Palgrave Studies in the Theory and History of Psychology

Series editor

Jack Martin
Department of Psychology
Simon Fraser University
Burnaby, BC
Canada

Palgrave Studies in the Theory and History of Psychology publishes scholarly books that use historical and theoretical methods to critically examine the historical development and contemporary status of psychological concepts, methods, research, theories, and interventions. The books in the series are characterised by an emphasis on the concrete particulars of psychologists' scientific and professional practices, together with a critical examination of the assumptions that attend their use. These examinations are anchored in clear, accessible descriptions of what psychologists do and believe about their activities. All the books in the series share the general goal of advancing the scientific and professional practices of psychology and psychologists, even as they offer probing and detailed questioning and critical reconstructions of these practices.

More information about this series at
http://www.springer.com/series/14576

Tom Strong

Medicalizing Counselling

Issues and Tensions

palgrave
macmillan

Tom Strong
University of Calgary
Calgary, BC
Canada

Palgrave Studies in the Theory and History of Psychology
ISBN 978-3-319-56698-6 ISBN 978-3-319-56699-3 (eBook)
DOI 10.1007/978-3-319-56699-3

Library of Congress Control Number: 2017938295

Printed on acid-free paper

This Palgrave Macmillan imprint is published by Springer Nature
The registered company is Springer International Publishing AG
The registered company address is: Gewerbestrasse 11, 6330 Cham, Switzerland

To counsellor education students, and the instructors supporting their journey. Your dedication to helping others through the conversational work you do has served as this book's inspiration.

Preface

Traditionally a field of widely contrasting and still-emerging approaches, counselling seems to be moving in step with a medicalizing mental health direction to address scientific legitimacy, financial administration, professional regulation, training, and other needs. Medicalization refers to a three-part logic: that human concerns are best understood as correctly diagnosable medical disorders, that these disorders require treatments proved efficient and effective in the same way expected of prescription medications, and that where diagnosed disorders are not treatable, they are manageable. Add to this logic that such disorders occur *in* people, relational or social justice issues are of little relevance, and people's strengths and resourcefulness are insignificant, and many counsellors can wonder what is becoming of their work should medicalization persist. Counselling has increasingly become synonymous, in the public's eyes, with mental health services, and for this service to be paid, this has meant counsellors being paid, managed, regulated, and approached by clients and colleagues as a health professional.

For many counsellors, this medicalizing direction will not be a problem, and helps to align their practice within mainstream mental health services. Needed for these counsellors is a common language to understand and address clients' concerns. Using DSM-5 diagnoses and evidence-based treatment honors scientific developments within psychiatry and psychology, while this language or discourse of mental health has clearly found its way into everyday understandings and conversations. However, medicalizing discourse is but one of the discourses that counsellors bring to conversations about clients' concerns and how to address them. Counsellors of all kinds have traditionally addressed client concerns in critically reflective, existential, relational, competency-eliciting, skill-developing or problem-solving, or social justice-focused ways. Counselling, in other words, has embraced a methodological pluralism comprising many approaches or discourses of practice—not all of which are compatible with a medicalizing discourse, or that will get them paid as professionals.

Critics of medicalization have for some time suggested that many formerly accepted aspects of the human condition have too quickly and too unproblematically been accepted as diagnosable medical conditions (e.g., bereavement, ADHD). Relatedly, critics of psychologization have suggested that human concerns are being reduced to individual, brain-based deficiencies, and are to be treated as such. Further, critics decry a pharmaceutical and technological direction that suggests our future quality of life will be best managed pharmaceutically or through new affective technologies. We are increasingly *governing* ourselves medically, say these critics. Counselling, in the face of these medicalizing developments, appears to be a modest helping practice. This book examines such critiques while advocating for a pluralistic conversational practice of counselling.

Approaching counselling as a conversational or discursive practice, I examine what I term medicalizing tensions. Medicalizing tensions refer to ways in which understandings and responses to human concerns are, in effect, competed for in the judgments of counsellors and the public making use of their services. Specifically, the conversations or precise communication protocols of medicalizing discourse can be at odds (or in tension) with the conversations by which non-medically oriented counsellors engage clients. There are aspects of counsellors' diverse approaches to conversational work that don't fit well with expected clinical algorithms based on medical diagnosis, treatment, and management. Frequently, counsellors take up different conversational foci depending on their discourse of practice, some seeming odd, medically speaking. Why focus on relational patterns, stories clients live by, unjust social circumstances, existential dilemmas, or client resourcefulness when there are mental disorders to be diagnosed and treated? Why see the relationship or the conversation as anything more than an information exchange? Counsellors have answers to such questions, answers that are often inconsistent with those taking a medicalized approach to their work.

Counselling has a relatively recent history of helping people overcome problems and difficulties that could, if unaddressed, become more serious mental health concerns. It also can be seen as part of a disappearing social safety net in an era of managed care and social service cuts. This book proposes we rethink what recent medicalizing developments have brought to counselling, and what could be lost if counselling develops further without its diverse approaches to helping others.

Calgary, Canada Tom Strong

Acknowledgements

I write these words of thanks during the holiday period of 2016/17. It seems a particularly challenging and still uncertain future ahead, with either a hard/soft Brexit, or with a "wrecking crew" Trump administration likely to further influence the kinds of tensions this book examines. Counselling services, in tough and recent times, have been one of the easier budget cuts, whether this is in public services, or of the health benefits rationed under private health-care plans. At the same time, there are, in Canada from where I write, crisis-level concerns for opioid overdoses, reconciliation with First Nations peoples who are addressing the effects of a harsh colonized recent history, and economic and employment uncertainty for a rapidly expanding class of people Guy Standing has referred to as "the precariat." On one hand, there has never been a greater need for counselling, while on the other such services may become inaccessible to the people needing them.

This is a book that draws on my counselling background in corrections, schools, public mental health, and private practice contexts in which I worked from the late 1970s to the end of the 1990s. To the many people I conversed with over those years—clients and colleagues—our conversations are sometimes refracted here, particularly with regard to how medicalization constrained us at times. To even recognize those constraints, however, it took my early 1990s exposure to Michael White to creatively and critically expand my sense of why discourse matters so much to the conversational work counsellors do. Other idea synthesizers took me further in this direction: Ken Gergen, Harlene Anderson, and Lois Holzman. I was lucky to have forged late 1990s internet connections to people who wanted to join me in furthering these important ideas: Andy Lock, David Paré, and Jerry Gale, who were great colleagues and writing partners, helped me make the big jump from practice to academic life.

I have found a good home base at the University of Calgary, which has enabled me to work with new colleagues (Karl Tomm, Dan Wulff, Sally St. George, Jeff Chang) a great group of postdocs (Monica Sesma-Vazquez and Gloria Dada Sanchez) and graduate students, many of whom have been patient collaborators as I was grappling with the kinds of ideas that went into this book. There are some particular students whose outstanding efforts have been crucial to me in completing this book: Konstantinos Chondros, Vanessa Vegter, and Karen Ross, but also Leah Beach, and Art Assoiants. In related ways, Inés Sametband, Tanya Mudry, Joaquín Gaete Silva, Jared French, Ottar Ness, Robbie Busch, Olga Sutherland, Don Zeman, and Shari Couture shared in many of the adventures and struggles that made up this journey. The research that helped to inform parts of this book was funded by the Social Sciences and Humanities Research Council of Canada as well as the University of Calgary. I have also been supported by some very understanding students and colleagues who sometimes had to go to great lengths to pull me away from computer screens, or things I was reading, as I was putting this book together.

Finally, as I was nearing completion of this book, a primary intellectual influence—John Shotter—passed away. I've been channeling John's influence here by translating his attention to the "cultural politics of everyday living" and "conversational realities" into these thoughts regarding the tensions medicalizing discourse poses for counselling. To my parents, who are clear beneficiaries of medicalization, may there be more years ahead of us.

Contents

List of Figures

1

Tensions in Medicalizing the Talking "Cure"

The irony of biological reductionism in psychology and psychiatry is that it is essentially an attempt to … use the "de-valued" language of the physical sciences to explain the value-laden (and "messy") world of human psychology from when they sprang in the first place.
(Thomas and Bracken 2011: 19)

A few years ago, I saw a client who came to me with what she described as debilitating anxiety attacks. When I asked her about when these attacks began, she spoke of an incident in the hospital where she worked, a hospital which had gone through major cutbacks in staffing. She worked overnight shifts alone from a nursing station situated to make access to patients in two wings accessible: geriatric as well as pediatric. Her resourceful solution to this challenging circumstance was to place babies in bassinettes on her nursing station desk, so that she could give them her primary attention, while attending to other patients' needs in both wings. One night, however, a geriatric patient went into cardiac arrest and during the time it took for other health professionals to join her, that geriatric patient died. It wasn't until she returned to her station and recognized that her other

T. Strong, *Medicalizing Counselling*, Palgrave Studies in the Theory and History of Psychology, DOI 10.1007/978-3-319-56699-3_1

vulnerable patients, the babies, had been without care for some time that her symptoms began. Rationally, she knew that she had not failed in her professionalism, so our conversation turned to the circumstance that had called her professionalism into question in the first place: the impossible staffing situation. My non-evidence-based treatment for her anxiety symptoms, so to speak, was to join in recognizing this circumstance, and to support her decision to involve her union in pressing the staffing issue.

Counselling tends to be sought for a wide range of concerns and aspirations, though that range has been narrowing, at least for privately and publicly funded counselling in our Canadian government-funded mental health services. While understood in various ways, counselling has been a changing repository of professional and cultural hopes for enhancing people's lives. Today, literally hundreds of approaches are practiced, while some from a few decades ago now seem quaint or dangerous. Despite this proliferation of approaches, most public and privately funded counselling has been narrowing to a medicalizing focus on diagnosable symptoms and treatable disorders. For the client mentioned there were diagnosable symptoms needing treatment, but our conversational work together also technically departed from the funded services for which she could see me.

I could have referred to many other clients and their concerns, as I saw them: the high school student determined to go to university but whose parents and religion expected otherwise, the family paralyzed with grief after a promising child developed a serious head injury, the client who became so fed up with his job he took a chainsaw to his leg, the couples who had lost their love, or clients who needed some way to "up periscope" and reflect on their priorities. With a poetic and ethical stretch, each client and concern could be probably be diagnosed and justified as medically meeting public service mandates and private funding criteria (e.g. Moses 2000; Pedowitz and Lustig 2014). However, it is just as likely that these concerns would not meet the requisite diagnostic criteria for funded counselling. The conversational work done in counselling with these clients wasn't treatment in a medical sense either.

Counselling, Tensions, Medicalizing Discourse, and Conversational Work

For our purposes, counselling will mean forms of conversational helping, professional conversations aimed to help others with varied human concerns and aspirations that have not always been seen as medical in nature. On first consideration, a single coherent approach to counselling—one that enables counsellors to effectively collaborate with other health-care professionals—seems a worthy goal. A medicalizing discourse of counselling, as I will be describing it, has been pursued as one such approach. The "ing" of medicaliz*ing* reflects an intent to refer to a past and still-unfolding process—the cultural phenomenon of medicalization. Standardizing the practice of counselling under a common medicalizing discourse of diagnosis, and evidence-based treatment for diagnosed conditions, has been shaping counsellors' practice over time, partly in response to changing mental health standards and administrative needs. Counselling should be offered on bases similar to other forms of health care goes the logic. The advances made by health scientists have been spectacular, resulting in longer and better-quality lives; counselling can be seen to benefit from such science, though views vary on those benefits.

To write of medicalizing discourse is to suggest that medicalization is one of many plausible discourses by which human concerns could be understood. Discourses, in this sense, are coherent systems of meaning by which people can communicate how they make sense of and address human concerns. For example, Brinkmann (2014) recently suggested that we frequently overlook that there are many discourses of suffering. Counselling approaches can also be understood as discourses (Paré 2013), as distinct ways to understand and respond to clients' concerns and hopes. For Hannah Arendt (1959), the human condition posed normal dilemmas and challenges such as aging or bereavement. These are concerns people formerly accepted, though, as diagnosable and treatable conditions, this assumption is shifting, so that we can now get on with lives that have less hassle and suffering. For example, diseases that shortened our lives are now treated as chronic conditions or disorders (e.g. diabetes; Clarke et al. 2010) to manage either biochemically or by other regimes of care. Medicalizing discourse has a diagnose-and-treat logic (Conrad 2007). Increasingly, the default language of self-understanding and self-determination, for media sociologist Eva Illouz (2008), is a medicalizing discourse underpinned by a medicalizing logic. By the time many clients show up in counselling this logic already has cued up particular understandings of their concerns and what should be done about them in counselling (Strong et al. 2015).

This translation of formerly accepted aspects of the human condition into treatable disorders has brought many improvements. In my own life, I can read with eyes that have had Lasik surgery, stay active because of a titanium knee, and benefit from anticoagulant medication for a clotting issue. These are quality of life-enhancing options that were unavailable two generations ago, and any fair assessment of medicalization should be conducted according to what it affords and constrains as life-enhancing possibilities (Gibson 1979). Enhancing the quality of our emotional and psychological lives through medicalizing developments has brought benefits but also some downsides (or tensions) we will examine.

Medicalizing tensions arise for counsellors accustomed to understanding and responding to client concerns using discourses of practice experienced as being at odds with medicalizing discourse. For many counsellors, client concerns do not always translate well to diagnosable disorders needing treatment. Counsellors, for example, who embrace family systems, meaning-oriented, or social justice-focused approaches, will make sense of client concerns in varied ways that raise such translation issues, or medicalizing tensions. Should sibling rivalry, disillusionment over one's vocation, or gender discrimination be diagnosed as mental disorders—such questions highlight translation issues or tensions counsellors might face. The tensions can develop further around the evidence-based "treatments" they may be expected to use. Counsellors have traditionally responded to client concerns that were considered non-psychiatric in severity, but in taking up roles within public mental health systems or through privately funded services, expected use of psychiatric or medicalizing discourse follows. How counsellors understand and reconcile tensions between their preferred approaches to practice and the "diagnose and treat" medicalizing discourse of mental health culture will be central to this book.

As Philip Cushman (1995) has shown, what has been diagnosable and treatable as psychiatric or psychologically disorders has been, to some degree, historically and culturally arbitrary. Medical or psychiatric science, Cushman argues, should be understood as being embedded within varying cultural and historical contexts where different notions of disease and disorder, as well as scientific methods, acquire significance and legitimacy. How medicalization works today may relate to an observation of David Morris (1998) about "postmodern illnesses" occurring where culture and biology intersect. Where, for example, does culture end and science begin when considering childhood misbehavior, grief, or career or marital dissatisfaction? What are we to make of the claims of Horwitz and Wakefield, that psychiatry has been transforming normal sadness into diagnosable depression (2007) or everyday fears into diagnosable anxiety (2012)? Answers to such questions speak to a sometimes confusing boundary between cultural expectations and what medical understandings and interventions can deliver. Even within psychiatry, excessive medicalization has been raised as a concern—enough for the editor of the *Diagnostic Manual of Mental Disorders: Fourth Edition* (DSM-IV, APA 1994; Frances 2013) to warn of expansionist tendencies in medicalizing normal aspects of the human condition, such as bereavement.

Counselling's relatively recent involvement with medicalizing discourse partly developed in tandem with research based on the diagnostic language of DSM-III in 1980 (APA 1980) and from changes in subsequent editions of the DSM, up to the present DSM-5 (APA 2013). Prior to the DSM-III, psychiatrists, as well as counsellors, were relatively inconsistent in how they made sense of clients' concerns, but the DSM-III's diagnostic criteria enabled a new clinical science requiring diagnostic precision from which "treatments" (first medications, then psychological interventions) could be evaluated. Thus, the rigors of the lab were expected to translate to understanding and addressing clients' concerns.

Such developments exemplify what Conrad referred to as the "shifting engines of medicalization" (Conrad 2007), and his 1970s studies of medicalization focused on a then new, but now culturally accepted, diagnosis: Attention Deficit and Hyperactivity Disorder (ADHD). My own schooldays predate Conrad's initial research; back then students in my classes were understood as fidgety, but not psychologically or psychiatrically disordered (see Nylund 2000). Since ADHD's diagnostic debut there has been an "epidemic" of sorts (see Frances 2013), as indicated by a recent study showing a fivefold increase in ADHD medication prescriptions in the decade between 1990 and 2001 (Dalsgaard et al. 2013). While we will visit the role of Big Pharma in medicalizing discourses as they relate counselling, it is also important to look at the way that the presumed expert knowledge of mental health professionals has found a receptive public who can learn about their concerns from accessible media (Illouz 2008; Jutel 2011). What shifted with medicalizing discourse were increasing client expectations that it become *the* legitimate language to discuss their concerns in counselling (Strong et al. 2015).

Counsellors have been adapting to medicalizing developments, particularly given how they have come to be seen as one of the professions that contributes to the public's mental health. How counselling came to be conflated with mental health services is part of the medicalizing story ahead. It is a story that is partly associated with the professional legitimacy psychological and medical science helped to confer, but also a story related to getting paid. While counsellors have typically left the more severe concerns some might consider medical with other professionals, like clinical psychologists and psychiatrists, they were also ambitious to expand their scope of practice. For example, when I began my training in the early 1980s, counsellors and therapists were typically seen as different professions, with the latter purportedly having more in-depth training and supervision in a particular approach to practice. Psychologists, since Rogers (1941), however, have tended to use both terms, though counsellors have been more circumspect. How the terms counsellor and therapist became interchangeable may have reflected a profession-legitimizing development, but it nudged things further in a medicalizing direction.

Counselling seems a modest professional activity when contrasted with the more official-sounding practice of psychotherapy. Evidently, many counsellors of the last generation thought so too. My Canadian Counselling Association (CCA) followed the British Association for Counselling (BAC), and upgraded its name to the Canadian Counselling and Psychotherapy Association (CCPA) (the BAC had upgraded to become the BACP in 2000—the "P" being for psychotherapy). One rationale offered was professional legitimacy, particularly for what equating counselling with psychotherapy could mean for members getting paid by public or private funders (CCPA, n.d.). As a counsellor educator, however, I still make this distinction, to convey a less medically oriented understanding of the counselling's conversational work, than, say, the work done by physical or respiratory therapists—though, yes, there are also have art and music therapists.

The notion of conversational work will be central to some of the distinctions and related tensions raised as we go forward. Counsellors' conversational work often begins with navigating and negotiating differences in discourse between clients and counsellors, and, at times, among colleagues, funders, and administrators. Counsellors using any discourse of practice tend to conceptualize and inquire into client concerns from premises consistent with their discourse(s), though they may respond to client concerns using several discourses of practice, including a medicalizing discourse. This is why the narrative counsellor listens for a problem-saturated client story, and evidence of a new client-preferred story, or why a feminist counsellor might focus on client oppression and opportunities for empowerment. Very different kinds of conversation occur as these discourses of practice conversationally engage clients and counsellors. A medicalizing conversation focused on diagnosing symptom clusters for later treatment differs from a solution-focused conversation regarding client strengths, preferences, and resourcefulness. Medicalizing tensions can arise for counsellors when what clients want from counselling won't meet requirements for an agency or funder's medicalizing discourse (e.g. a relational or vocational problem). Clients bring their own discourses of understanding that can be worth reflecting upon and altering, and they may already be schooled in medicalizing discourse themselves.

Counselling's conversation work gets differently accounted for depending on the metaphors of communication used to inform that work (Lakoff and Johnson 1980; Turnbull 2003). For example, some counselling approaches, and medicine more generally, approach language as a means to correctly represent and understand experience, with conversation being how such understandings are transmitted and received. This is not the view of communication I will bring to this critical review; however, such a view also relates to the medicalizing tensions we will consider. With the added sensitivities to discourse brought by Foucault (1973) and early microanalyses of therapeutic discourse (e.g. Labov and Fanshel 1977; Scheflen 1973) came challenges to the notion that the conversational work of counselling was about information exchanges or directives, requiring counsellors to communicate correctly. For many counsellors, counselling is a meaning-making activity where meaning and conversational process is negotiated in ways difficult to prescribe. Standardizing the language of counselling, to be consistent with that used by other mental health professions is another medicalizing tension counsellors can experience.

Scientific Discourses and Counselling

No discourse addresses everything relevant to the concerns and aspirations clients bring to counselling, and this should not be seen as a failing of medical or psychological science (Gergen 2005). Differences in discourse cannot be resolved with value-neutral science, and that is what Thomas and Bracken were getting at in this chapter's opening quotation. Many client concerns could be understood as conflicts where different values are relevant to resolution of the concerns. Some of the tensions we will visit relate to the science–practice divide where differences in values are very much in play. This, however, has not stopped people from people considering how science could put their concerns behind them. If you have ever wondered if medical or psychological science could tell me how I should live my life, you may have encountered some of these tensions, particularly if you have read some Foucault (2003).

Referring to such medicalizing developments as occurring within a specific discourse is important for drawing attention to medicalizing as a social process and social construction (Burr 2003). Discourses, as such, have been equated with ideologies, with those most worthy of critical attention usually being already operative in our lives in taken-for-granted ways (Eagleton 1991). How medicalization has become interwoven with counselling as well as people's everyday lives prompts some of the reflection here. Medicalization developed as a focus of critical sociological interest after Zola (1972) drew attention to how its expert-based influence was expanding into new aspects of human life, for better and worse. His interest arose around the same time Foucault (1973) brought attention to the spaces and practices he associated with "medical perception." Twinning this perception with addressing what had previously been understood as moral, spiritual, and existential challenges enabled such challenges to be recast as psychological or psychiatric problems to be diagnosed, treated, and managed (Danziger 1997).

One illustrative example of what I mean by the taken-for-grantedness of social constructions can be found when reflecting upon how time has been humanly constructed. Harvard historian of science, Peter Galison (2004), chronicled the great debates that went into *negotiating* the 24-h world clock. This was a development that seemed unrequired until technology, such as telegraph communications, advanced to the point that it became clear that breakfast-time correspondence from New York did not amount to the same in San Francisco. In the end, the solution was part science and part political negotiation between nations. The upshot is that the world's technologies could be coordinated by this humanly constructed world clock, that still produced imperfections like the International Date Line and a much later Y2K scare based on how time was programmed into computer technology. Our humanity is transformed by such constructions and their technological applications, and such is the case with medicalization.

Examining how our humanity became interwoven (or "entangled"; Barad 2007) with such technological and other material aspects of life in taken-for-granted ways is central to this book's storyline. With medicalization has come new knowledge and technologies with a bearing on both personal well-being and counselling, which we will examine through the critical lens afforded by science and technology scholars (e.g. Latour 2005, 2013). For these scholars, we become transformed by our human constructions; whether they are new discourses, technologies, or even forms of mental health hygiene. A particular institutional culture has followed from developments associated with medicalizing discourse: mental health. Foucaultian scholars, like Rose, have termed one version of this culture the "psy-complex," to draw attention to how psychological science and its applications have been shaping, for some time, our conceptions of selfhood, self-care, and care of others (see Rose 1985, 1990). Critiquing this entanglement of medicalized knowledge and technology should not be confused with being anti-scientific, so it is important to address this concern before going further.

Key to any science are the very human activities that Ian Hacking (1983) has referred to as "representing and intervening." When these activities produce knowledge and results through careful, rigorous, peer-reviewed science, what matters is that the resulting knowledge can be effectively used. Effective knowledge is correct in the sense that it produces intended results or applications, like smartphones or medical breakthroughs. However, there is no sense that such effective knowledge can be claimed as ultimately or universally correct, as I hope this next example helps to illustrate. If brought together to explain and create laughter, a biochemist, an anthropologist, a neuroscientist, and a linguist could offer their respective disciplines' best knowledge—but who is correct? The question is a distraction, for each scientist arguably has something useful to say, but on the basis of very different discourses (see Latour 2013). Much of mental health is grounded in a single scientific discourse (DSM-5) for the concerns clients bring. It is a discourse that the United States' National Institute of Mental Health (NIMH) indicated it will no longer fund research purposes (April 29, 2013), turning instead to a neuroscientific discourse (Insel 2013).

Social sciences were arguably turned to for the same kinds of knowledge that put an astronaut on the moon, or that keeps making "smarter" devices; but humans aren't like plants, planets, or other non-sentient features of the environment. In step with cultural and historical developments, our concerns, over, say, substance "misuse," can vary (Cushman 1995), and so can the language we use to describe our concerns (Danziger 1997). Some of the struggle that can be associated with what I am raising can come down to a distinction made by the hermeneutic scholar, Gadamer (1988); namely, that, when accounting for humans we can understand (using whatever discourse we might employ to do so) but never fully explain. Medicalizing discourse will be therefore approached as a way of partially understanding and responding to human concerns, while recognizing that, with other counselling discourses, what matters is its effective use in addressing concerns clients might bring to counselling.

Mental Health Culture: Where Psychological and Medical Discourses Converge

Mental health has become what others, borrowing from Deleuze, term an assemblage (Duff 2014), and counselling arguably has become increasingly interwoven within that assemblage. In other words, counselling has increasingly become administered according to particular accountabilities that link science-informed front-line practice to administrative practice occurring at a distance. Thus, an assemblage can be a bureaucratic, machine-like, institutional culture that has material consequences for those caught up in its processes, discourse, and logic. To obtain counselling or provide it brings entanglements with mental health administration requirements for accountable practice—for client as well as counsellor. How or even if counselling occurs involves far more than the counsellor and client's decision-making. The same could be said about their conversations, which are ostensibly rationed and supervised according to particular algorithms associated with diagnosed conditions and evidence-based treatments.

Such algorithms or protocols for managing mental health require psychiatry's DSM-5 diagnoses, but also psychology's clinical science. Counselling, however, has had a complicated relationship with psychology. To what extent counselling requires the application of psychological knowledge is a question we will consider, particularly reflecting upon the psy-complex of Rose (1985). Most counsellor education programs are informed by diverse forms of psychological knowledge and principles of practice, found in the strikingly different approaches of counselling theories textbooks such as those by McLeod (2013) or Corey

(2016). Counselling, like counselling psychology, however, has had an inferiority complex when contrasted with its emulated elder sibling, clinical psychology (Ogunfowora and Drapeau 2008), despite it helping to address concerns that could become psychopathology (Zimmer-Gembeck and Skinner 2016).

Psychology has been cozy with medicine for some time, largely for sharing a similar logic of practice, but like psychiatry it had to overcome some public perception issues. Central to legitimizing psychological practice—for funding and public perception purposes—has been the development of evidence-based practice (EBP) often equated with evidence-based medicine (Dobson 2016). Tethering this evidence-based approach to practice is the diagnostic language of the DSM and this, among other reasons, has sparked great debates within psychology (Levant 2005; Levittet al., 2005; Wampold et al. 2005). These debates can seem remote to the average counsellor or student of counselling until they seek employment or practicum opportunities, as mental *health* professionals (Strong et al. 2017).

There has been considerable criticism of this medicalizing direction for counselling. Early critiques of mental health (Goffman 1961; Ingleby 1980) largely focused on institutional abuses of patients. But another critique grew out of concerns regarding psychology's normative, individualizing, and essentializing science—particularly regarding how the science was to be applied in such professional services as education and counselling (Henriques et al. 1984). At first glance, a medicalized approach, backed by psychological science, would seem to exemplify a kind of scientific Darwinism at work; through scientific trial and error, other approaches were deservedly consigned to counselling's scrap heap.

No question, counselling has seen some odd and harmful approaches that skeptics are quick to point out: primal scream therapy, naked encounter groups, and so on. The contemporary science of counselling and counselling interventions, however, continuously yields one solid conclusion: that it is the quality of the counselling relationship or conversational work that matters most (Duncan et al. 2010). The interventions of counselling cannot be equated with pharmaceutical interventions (Stiles and Shapiro 1989); nor can clients' varied responses to counselling interventions be ignored (Kramer and Stiles 2015). In other words, counselling tends to be understood as a relational or conversational practice first, and, secondarily, as a practice requiring adherence to specific diagnostic or intervention procedures, as is the case in a medicalizing approach or discourse of practice.

I am a counselling *psychologist* so it might seem odd that I relate the medicalizing tensions I will be detailing to too great a focus on individual problems associated with the psyche. Like many drawn to psychology, my initial motivation was to find out what made people "tick" so that I would understand how to help when things weren't ticking so well. Human concerns brought to counselling had causes and solutions; my job was to learn these causes and solutions and focus my conversations with clients accordingly. Presumably, the applied knowledge of psychology should be like the standardized knowledge used by engineers and doctors. My personal concern about this medicalizing logic of science-backed choices (cf. Mol 2008) initially developed during my training in family systems approaches in the 1980s, but grew as postmodern, multicultural, and linguistic philosophy issues became more familiar to me.

Following a decade of front-line counselling, in the late 1990s I returned to university life, in part because of concerns that played a role in motivating my writing this book. I had embraced discursive approaches to counselling (narrative, solution-focused, collaborative, see Lock and Strong 2012; Strong and Paré 2004), but was rubbing up against how developments in researching, training, and administering counselling had failed to support these counselling approaches. Part of the issue was the diagnosis-based psychological and medical science that had accelerated in the late 1990s and early 2000s. An evidence-based approach for evaluating psychological interventions had been imported from the Cochrane Collaboration, which focused on effective and efficient health services (http://www.cochrane.org/about-us/our-name).

Having counselled in both publicly and privately funded contexts, my experience of medicalizing discourse hadn't been much of a problem; I practiced using my preferred systemic and discursively informed approaches. This wasn't, however, the experience of my colleague, Dr. Karl Tomm, a psychiatrist well known for his contributions to family therapy, whose primary focus has been on addressing problematic family patterns of interaction. While always clear on avoiding an either/or focus (i.e. individual versus family well-being), he was once told that the internationally renowned Calgary Family Therapy Centre he directed was required to use DSM diagnoses. Behind this requirement were expectations for accountability within the provincially funded health services system. Tomm's response, almost 25 years ago, was to develop a family systems assessment system used to assess and monitor family functioning, and his Centre's provincial funding has been based on that system ever since (Tomm et al. 2014). My point here is not to advocate for another system of assessment and intervention in counselling, but to highlight discursive alternatives for addressing tensions over administrative and professional expectations associated with a medicalizing discourse.

Part of my motivation in writing this book is to raise concerns about a narrowing of discursive options for the important work counsellors do. I recall an interview I did over a decade ago with then National Geographic Explorer in residence, Wade Davis and Tom Strong (2003), regarding his study of cultural healing practices. Davis had studied voodoo culture and healing practices on the Amazon while completing his Harvard doctorate in Anthropology. Davis spoke of an "ethnosphere" comprising the planet's diverse forms of healing wisdom, wisdoms rooted in the ways cultures communicate (i.e. discourses) that were rapidly disappearing. For him, that put the planet at risk, that "progress" associated with this downside of modernity could undermine our ways of understanding and responding to threats to our common humanity. I similarly approach the many discourses of counselling as offering resources that make different contributions to understanding and responding to our concerns. Secondarily, I think a critical awareness of how discourses, like medicalizing discourse, operate so as to constrain discursive resourcefulness (see Strong 2016) is a key feature of what I hope to explore as you read on.

Going forward, Chap. 2 explicates and historically traces a discursive view of counselling. By discursive, I elaborate on two primary notions: that counselling occurs through discourse, and that many discourses can be reflected upon and productively used in counselling. A lot goes missing from what counselling is or could be if medicalizing discourse dominates how counselling comes to be understood and practiced. Counselling clearly can make differences in people's lives, regardless of whether it is understood as a medical or allied health service (Seligman 2004). However, medicalization is not a benign discourse for professionals and others who understand and undertake counselling on pluralistic terms. Specifically, counsellors, students of counselling, counsellor educators, counselling organizations, and the service-seeking public have all had to contend with influences of medicalizing discourse.

Chapter 3 focuses on the development and implications of psychiatry's diagnostic discourse (DSM-5). Understanding the concerns prospective clients might present in counselling as diagnosable symptom clusters needing medical treatment is a longstanding practice. However, as expectations for its use by counsellors grow, other discourses and approaches to practice can seem incompatible with that use. For example, how do social injustices, existential crises, or relational challenges (also concerns brought to counsellors)—get responded to in a society that narrows its helping services to diagnosable disorders warranting medical treatment? Such questions speak to the tensions I will be associating with medicalization and counselling, but also relate to cultural developments (Illouz 2008) associated with how people have come to understand and medicalize themselves and the "human condition."

Chapter 4 explores the notion that counselling may, to legitimize itself, have overcommitted to a mental health monoculture. While they may not wear stethoscopes, in the public imagination counsellors have come to be seen as part of the continuum of services one associates with health care and medicine. This is despite a professed pluralism of counselling traditions or discourses inconsistent with this logic from many counsellors (Cooper and McLeod 2011). This kind of pluralism refers to the many traditions and discourses (i.e. approaches) used by counsellors, only some of which fit within the medicalizing (diagnose and treat) logic and discourse I have been describing. How a mental health monoculture has developed and what the resultant tensions might mean for counselling is Chap. 4's focus.

Chapter 5 examines an implication of medicalization that has prompted considerable critical reflection for counsellors; namely, that a medically focused counselling directs attention away from social justice, existential, relational, and other formulations of clients' concerns. In other words, a medicalizing approach focused on diagnosing and treating individual symptoms could bypass the aid central to how counsellors self-identify as professionals, through their varied counselling discourses. For example, when might one person's presumed depression be alternatively understood as oppression? Has a medicalizing mental health focus also been promoted by popular media, prompting some critics to decry ours as a "therapeutic culture" (Furedi 2004) having made a "therapeutic turn" (Madsen 2014). What these developments mean for counselling, and our increasingly neoliberal society, will focus this chapter's focus on the implications of a potential, dominant mental health monoculture.

Chapter 6 examines relatively recent tensions associated with society's (and counselling's) increasing use of medicalizing technologies and pharmaceutical treatments. One aspect of these tensions comes with how the discourse and logic of medicalization has increasingly been technologically embedded into self-help culture—from personal apps to cyber-blogs and pharmaceuticalization. Medicalizing logic has become central to identities and self-management strategies brought by clients to counsellors. Another focus will be on the role that medications now have in the lives of clients and for the conversational work of counselling. This chapter tackles perhaps the most recognizable aspect of medicalization, and technology that is only beginning to get on our radar (Braidotti 2013; Clarke et al. 2010).

Chapter 7 brings readers into the professional debates associated with the administration of counselling on medicalizing terms. Perhaps more than any other influence, the funding and administration of counselling has propelled counselling further into a situation that now merits critical reflection. Medicalization (DSM-5 and EBPs) offers administrators a way to manage and ration counselling as a practice, while further enabling counselling's alignment with other mental health professions where arguably counsellors can join other differently trained professionals as "therapists." Professionally, counselling associations and organizations have had to carefully position themselves to respond to member preferences, governmental statutes, and marketplace realities. Professionally and administratively counsellors face medicalizing tensions now that were not part of practice a generation ago, and this chapter examines these tensions.

Chapter 8 focuses on counsellors in the front lines of practice; how medicalizing tensions are experienced, and how they navigate and negotiate these tensions in their everyday work with clients, colleagues, and administrators. I will be drawing on two prior studies (Strong et al. 2012, forthcoming-b) that involved surveys and interviews with counsellors, counsellor educators, and profession leaders who spoke at length about these tensions. At times, I will zoom out to talk about the contexts in which these tensions are experienced while at other times I will zoom into focus on the conversational work reported to us. The aim of this chapter is to situate counsellors, and those interested in counselling, into how medicalization plays out in the conversational work and institutional requirements that engage counsellors.

Chapter 9 takes us into experiences and debates shaping the next generation of counsellors: the graduate students and recent graduates of counsellor education programs. It is in university settings where the research and professional leadership shaping the future of counselling can be found, and we will examine some of the ways this future-building is occurring. We will also examine the role that critical and discursive approaches to psychology play in counsellor education, extending the recent focus given to social justice issues (e.g., for minority and vulnerable clients).

Chapter 10 will pull together the earlier chapters in ways that both summarize the medicalizing tensions for counselling while returning to a theme that I associate with discursive awareness and discursive resourcefulness (Strong 2016). I will approach this chapter as a plea to the profession to not narrow its practice focus to diagnosing and treating client symptoms but to continue to advocate for its pluralistic traditions and future innovations that may be incompatible with medicalization. Bottom line, I will advocate that important leadership is needed to retain counselling as a distinct professional activity (though I agree it can be done by other professions) without constraining it solely to a medical approach.

This is a book that I hope invites further dialogue and reflection on what I have been describing as a medicalizing discourse of counselling. While counselling and psychotherapy have sometimes been referred to as the "talking cure" (Cushman 1995), making medicalizing discourse sound like counselling's first language, we will be considering it as one of many discourses of practice. The counselling examined here has traditions that focus on everyday concerns or Szasz's (1961) problems in living. There has long been an aspect of counselling that could be seen as part of society's safety net, and in lots of ways counsellors make differences in clients' lives. Symptom relief is certainly part of those differences. Counsellors have also, however, provided assistance in aspects of life not so well encompassed by a medicalizing view. They are interested in helping clients navigate and negotiate the value-laden and messy worlds Thomas and Bracken (2011) described in this chapter's opening quote. In my view, there are lots of ways to help clients with that navigating and negotiating that won't neatly fit under one umbrella called mental health or medicalization. That belief is where the tensions I will be describing arises from, and by the book's end I hope to invite greater consideration of that belief.

References

APA (American Psychiatric Association). (1980). *Diagnostic and statistical manual of mental disorders* (3rd ed.). Washington: Author.

APA (American Psychiatric Association). (1994). *Diagnostic and statistical manual of mental disorders* (4th ed.). Washington: Author.

APA (American Psychiatric Association). (2013). *Diagnostic and statistical manual of mental disorders* (5th ed.). Washington: Author.

Arendt, H. (1959). *The human condition.* Garden City, NY: Doubleday Anchor.

Barad, K. (2007). *Meeting the universe halfway: Quantum physics and the entanglement of matter and meaning.* Durham, NC: Duke University Press.

Braidotti, R. (2013). *The Posthuman.* Cambridge: Polity Press.

Brinkmann, S. (2014). Languages of suffering. *Theory & Psychology, 24*(5), 630–648.

Burr, V. (2003). *Social constructionism* (2nd ed.). New York: Routledge.

Clarke, A. E., Mamo, L., Fosket, J. R., Fishman, J. R., & Shim, J. K. (Eds.). (2010). *Biomedicalization: Technoscience, health and illness in the US.* Durham, NC: Duke University Press.

Conrad, P. (2007). *The medicalization of society*. Baltimore: Johns Hopkins University Press.

Cooper, M., & McLeod, J. (2011). *Pluralistic counselling and psychotherapy*. Thousand Oaks, CA: Sage.

Corey, G. (2016). *Theory and practice of counseling and psychotherapy* (10th ed.). Boston: Cengage Learning.

Cushman, P. (1995). *Constructing the self, constructing America: A cultural history of psychotherapy*. Boston: Da Capo Press.

Dalsgaard, S., Nielsen, H. S., & Simonsen, M. (2013). Five-fold increase in national prevalence rates of attention-deficit/hyperactivity disorder medication for children and adolescents with autism spectrum disorder, attention-deficit/hyperactivity disorder, and other psychiatric disorders: A Danish register-based study. *Journal of Child and Adolescent Psychopharmacology, 23*(7), 432–439.

Danziger, K. (1997). *Naming the mind: How psychology found its language*. Thousand Oaks, CA: Sage.

Davis, W., & Strong, T. (2003, September/October). Healing culture. *New Therapist*, 27, 10–17.

Dobson, K. S. (2016). Clinical psychology in Canada: Challenges and opportunities. *Canadian Psychology, 57*(3), 211–219.

Duff, C. (2014). *Assemblages of health: Deleuze's empiricism and the ethology of life*. London: Springer.

Duncan, B. L., Miller, S. D., Wampold, B. E., & Hubble, M. A. (Eds.). (2010). *The heart and soul of change: Delivering what works in therapy* (2nd ed.). Washington: American Psychological Association.

Eagleton, T. (1991). *Ideology: An introduction*. New York: Verso.

Foucault, M. (1973). *The birth of the clinic: An archaeology of medical perception*. London: Tavistock.

Foucault, M. (2003). *Psychiatric power: Lectures at the collège de France, 1973–1974*. New York: Picador.

Frances, A. (2013). *Saving normal: An insider's revolt against out-of-control psychiatric diagnosis, DSM-5, big pharma, and the medicalization of ordinary life*. New York: William Morrow.

Furedi, F. (2004). *Therapy culture: Cultivating vulnerability in an uncertain age*. New York: Routledge.

Gadamer, H. G. (1988). *Truth and method* (2nd Rev. ed, J. Weinsheimer & D. G. Marshall, Trans.). London: Continuum.

Galison, P. (2004). *Einstein's clocks and Poincare's maps: Empires of time*. New York: W.W. Norton.

Gergen, K. J. (2005). *Therapeutic realities: Collaboration, oppression and relational flow*. Chagrin Falls, OH: Taos Institute Publications.

Gibson, J. J. (1979). *The ecological approach to visual perception*. London: Lawrence Erlbaum Associates.

Goffman, I. (1961). *Asylums: Essays on the social situation of mental patients and other inmates*. New York: Doubleday Anchor.

Hacking, I. (1983). *Representing and intervening: Introductory topics in the philosophy of natural science*. Cambridge: Cambridge University Press.

Henriques, J., Hollway, W., Urwin, C., Venn, C., & Walkerdine, V. (Eds.). (1984). *Changing the subject: Psychology, social regulation and subjectivity*. London: Methuen.

Horwitz, A. V., & Wakefield, J. C. (2007). *The loss of sadness: How psychiatry transformed normal sorrow into depressive disorder*. New York: Oxford University Press.

Horwitz, A. V., & Wakefield, J. C. (2012). *All we have to fear: Psychiatry's transformation of natural anxieties into medical disorders*. New York: Oxford University Press.

Illouz, E. (2008). *Saving the modern soul: Therapy, emotions, and the culture of self-help*. Berkeley: University of California Press.

Ingleby, D. (Ed.). (1980). *Critical psychiatry: The politics of mental health*. New York: Pantheon Books.

Insel, T. (2013). *Post by former NIMH director Thomas Insel: Transforming diagnosis*. Retrieved November 18, 2016, from https://www.nimh.nih.gov/about/directors/thomas-insel/blog/2013/transforming-diagnosis.shtml.

Jutel, A. G. (2011). *Putting a name to it: Diagnosis in contemporary society*. Baltimore: Johns Hopkins University Press.

Kramer, U., & Stiles, W. B. (2015). The responsiveness problem in psychotherapy: A review of proposed solutions. *Clinical Psychology: Science and Practice, 22*(3), 277–295.

Labov, W., & Fanshel, D. (1977). *Therapeutic discourse: Psychotherapy as conversation*. New York: Academic Press.

Lakoff, G., & Johnson, M. (1980). *Metaphors we live by*. Chicago: University of Chicago Press.

Latour, B. (2005). *Reassembling the social: An introduction to actor-network-theory*. Oxford: Oxford University Press.

Latour, B. (2013). *An inquiry into modes of existence: An anthropology of the moderns*. Cambridge, MA: Harvard University Press.

Levant, R. F. (2005). *Report of the 2005 presidential task force on evidence-based practice*. American Psychological Association. Accessed from https://www.apa.org/practice/resources/evidence/evidence-based-report.pdf.

Levitt, H. M., Neimeyer, R. A., & Williams, D. C. (2005). Rules versus principles in psychotherapy: Implications of the quest for universal guidelines in the movement for empirically supported treatments. *Journal of Contemporary Psychotherapy, 35*(1), 117–129.

Lock, A., & Strong, T. (Eds.). (2012). *Discursive perspectives in therapeutic practice*. New York: Oxford University Press.

Madsen, O. J. (2014). *The therapeutic turn: How psychology altered western culture*. New York: Routledge.

McLeod, J. (2013). *An introduction to counselling* (5th ed.). Maidenhead: Open University Press.

Mol, A. (2008). *The logic of care: Health and the problem of patient choice*. London: Routledge.

Morris, D. B. (1998). *Illness and culture in the postmodern age*. Berkeley: University of California Press.

Moses, I. (2000). Is it ethical to deceive managed care companies? A panel of the new editors of the journal of contemporary psychotherapy. *Journal of Contemporary Psychotherapy, 30*(3), 217–237.

Nylund, D. (2000). *Treating huckleberry finn: A new narrative approach with kids diagnosed ADD/ADHD*. San Francisco: Jossey-Bass.

Ogunfowora, B., & Drapeau, M. (2008). Comparing counselling and clinical psychology professionals: Similarities and differences on theoretical orientations revisited. *International Journal for the Advancement of Counselling, 30*(2), 93–103.

Paré, D. (2013). *The practice of collaborative counseling and psychotherapy: Developing skills in culturally mindful helping*. Los Angeles: Sage.

Pedowitz, R. T., & Lustig, S. L. (2014). Medical necessity review: History, innovation, and missed opportunity. *Psychiatric Times, 31*(6), 32.

Rogers, C. (1941). *Counseling and psychotherapy: Newer concepts in practice*. New York: Houghton Mifflin.

Rose, N. (1985). *The psychological complex: Psychology, politics and society in England, 1869–1939*. London: Routledge.

Rose, N. (1990). *Governing the soul: The shaping of the private self*. New York: Routledge.

Scheflen, A. E. (1973). *Communicational structure: Analysis of a psychotherapy transaction*. Bloomington: Indiana University Press.

Seligman, L. (2004). *Diagnosis and treatment planning in counseling* (3rd ed.). New York: Springer.

Stiles, W. B., & Shapiro, D. A. (1989). Abuse of the drug metaphor in psychotherapy process-outcome research. *Clinical Psychology Review, 9*(4), 521–543.

Strong, T. (2016). Discursive awareness and resourcefulness: Bringing discursive researchers into closer dialogue with discursive therapists? In M. O'Reilly & J. Lester (Eds.), *Adult mental health: Discourse and conversation studies*. London: Palgrave Macmillan.

Strong, T., & Paré, D. (2004). *Furthering talk: Advances in the discursive therapies*. New York: Kluwer Academic/Plenum.

Strong, T., Gaete, J., Sametband, I. N., French, J., & Eeson, J. (2012). Counsellors respond to the DSM-IV-TR. *Canadian Journal of Counselling and Psychotherapy, 46*(2), 85–106.

Strong, T., Ross, K. H., & Sesma-Vazquez, M. (2015). Counselling the (self?) diagnosed client: Generative and reflective conversations. *British Journal of Guidance and Counselling, 43*(5), 598–610.

Strong, T., Chondros, K., Job, C., & Vegter, V. (2017). Medicalizing Developments in Counsellor Education? Counselling and Counselling Psychology Students' Views. *Canadian Journal of Counselling and Psychotherapy, 57*, 161–186.

Strong, T., Chondros, K., Vegter, V., & Job, C. (forthcoming-b). Medicalizing tensions in counsellor education? *European Journal of Psychotherapy and Counselling*.

Szasz, T. (1961). *The myth of mental illness: Foundations of a theory of personal conduct*. New York: Hoeber-Harper.

Thomas, P., & Bracken, P. (2011). Dualisms and the myth of mental illness. In M. Rapley, J. Moncrieff, & J. Dillon (Eds.), *De-medicalizing misery: Psychiatry, psychology, and the human condition* (pp. 10–26). London: Palgrave Macmillan.

Tomm, K., St. George, S., Wulff, D., & Strong, T. (Eds.). (2014). *Patterns in interpersonal interactions: Inviting relational understandings for therapeutic change*. New York: Routledge.

Turnbull, W. (2003). *Language in action: Psychological models of conversation*. New York: Psychology Press.

Wampold, B. E., Lichtenberg, J. W., & Waehler, C. A. (2005). A broader perspective: Counseling psychology's emphasis on evidence. *Journal of Contemporary Psychotherapy, 35*(1), 27–38.

Zimmer-Gembeck, M. J., & Skinner, E. A. (2016). The development of coping: Implications for psychopathology and resilience. *Developmental Psychopathology, 4*(10), 1–61.

Zola, I. K. (1972). Medicine as an institution of social control. *The Sociological Review, 20,* 487–504.

2

Discourses of Counselling and Human Concern

[E]ssential to an experience is that it cannot be exhausted in what can be said of it or grasped as its meaning.
(Gadamer 1988: 67)

To suggest that counselling is best understood as discursive activity is not to diminish what can be at stake, for client and counsellor, in its conversational work. An ongoing challenge in counselling relates to how to regard the language used by clients and counsellors and what that use configures in terms of understandings, actions, and relationships. The heart of the challenge rests with recognizing that our concerns and actions do not name themselves; we do, in humanly constructed and variable languages, or discourses. The languages or discourses for concerns brought to counselling today convey origins and understandings that can challenge any shared sense of meaning. While counselling's words and language may vary, so too do our value-based meanings and the actions that follow from them. That is where notions of discourse come in. This chapter will focus on why discourse matters to counsellors, and why efforts to constrain its diversity, such as by medicalizing meanings and actions related to them, can be problematic.

T. Strong, *Medicalizing Counselling*, Palgrave Studies in the Theory and History of Psychology, DOI 10.1007/978-3-319-56699-3_2

Discourse, in one way I will use the term, refers to distinct systems or logics of meaning and informed action, like the discourse I have been calling medicalization. Such discourses operate like reality tunnels, as discrete ways of understanding, evaluating, and conducting life. At worst, that means one person's or group's reality is meaningfully walled off from the realities of others, because the linguistically based understandings of such realities are so different. One can stand back from patterns in such ways of understanding, communicating, and acting, and find a coherence that can be named, such as one might by identifying a discourse as patriarchy or globalization (Fairclough 1992). Inside such discourses, such meanings and logics often seem self-evident to those used to living by them. From outside, discourse patterns can be identified for how distinctly used words and logic cohere in recognizable systems of meaning. Along these lines, Wittgenstein (1953) wrote about how knowing a language (or discourse) can be like knowing a form of life. Counselling's pluralistic approaches to practice exemplify what I mean by discourses (Cooper and McLeod 2011; Paré 2013). Generally speaking, differences between discourses of counselling, or the counsellors taking these discourse up, have not been an issue.

There is another aspect of discourse central to our considerations. Discourse also refers to how communicative interaction occurs, how life gets navigated and negotiated between people, such as counsellors and clients. Discursively *navigating* life suggests uses of language to understand and address accepted realities, while discursively *negotiating* such realities can mean transforming such realities. Navigating and negotiating will be terms that help to identify the discursive tensions associated with this book's discursive view, terms we will revisit when considering how language gets *used* in counselling's conversational work.

Discourse can be confusing for having the two meanings described. On one hand it is noun-like, referring to distinct systems of meaning; while on the other, it is verb-like, referring to communicative interactions. For our purposes, I will usually refer to discourses in noun-like ways, such as when I describe medicalizing, neuroscience, or other discourses of counselling. However, the discursive or conversational work of counselling between clients and counsellors is where the tensions I will describe as medicalizing tensions will be central. The situated uses of discourse (medicalizing discourse and others) influence (cf. Mills 1940) and inform how people navigate and negotiate what occurs in the conversational or discursive work between them.

Referring to counselling's discursive work as involving navigations and negotiations of meaning can seem odd. By a critical view of discourse, negotiations, like those between a client and counsellor, are tilted to favor professional and institutional sources of power (Peräkylä et al. 2008; Rose 1990). This is especially the case with expert discourses (Abbott 1988), like medicalizing discourse, where roles like "patient" or health-care "provider" find clear definitions. Not all counselling approaches adopt this expert-based view of dialogue between counsellors and clients, and among narrative, solution-focused, collaborative, and feminist counsellors' client-centeredness is often focal (Proctor 2002). This privileging of client meanings has also sometimes been translated to a practical focus on client preferences and untapped client expertise (Anderson and Goolishian 1992), though the extent to which counsellors can share power in their dialogues has been a source of debate among discursive counsellors (Monk and Gehart 2003). Negotiating conversational meanings and processes with clients—meanings and processes they invest themselves in—is no small challenge for counsellors ready to acknowledge how discourses influence such meanings and processes (cf. Strong 2002). Tensions arise in how discourses, such as medicalizing discourse, influence clients' and counsellors' choice of words and conversational turn-taking.

Science and Discourses in Counselling?

A common view of professional discourse is that any profession's current language and meanings reflects the outcomes of a Darwinian struggle settled by science. Science, accordingly, should resolve tensions since these would-be anomalies seem to need a better evidence-informed explanation (Kuhn 1962). Prior or alternative meanings and language, by this logic, should most appropriately be consigned to any profession's linguistic and conceptual scrap heap. Therefore, students of counselling's history can derisively read about magic, "quaint" spiritual practices, or quack cures (Ehrenwald 1991) as part of the profession's embarrassing past. Critics, like Foucault (1968), Danziger (1997), or Cushman (1995), highlighted how varied historical understandings have been when making sense of and addressing human concerns. The notion that help for human concerns required professional expertise beyond a friend's or elder's wisdom and compassion is recent, if one looks beyond spiritual helping practices, such as confession. So, how is it that so many distinctive discourses developed within counselling? More to this chapter's point, how did a medicalizing discourse become so influential on counselling today?

Apart from sociologists, few scholars and professionals discuss science-informed professional counselling in discursive terms. The Tower of Babel is sometimes invoked when reflecting upon the different understandings and professional communications informing counselling discourses and approaches (e.g. Miller et al. 1997). A single, scientifically informed discourse of practice would seem an obvious answer to an unruly pluralism or dubious professional eclecticism. Still, counselling today continues to be learned using multiple discourses (cf. Heaton 2014), while efforts to standardize counselling under one professional discourse, medicalized or other, seem to generate profession-centered "tensions" (House 2004). Some of these tensions relate to how any discourse is partial in what it accounts for; something relevant seems inevitably left out of any discourse of counselling (Cecchin et al. 1992). So counsellors add new understandings; extending traditional discourses (or developing new ones) to account for concerns like cyber-pornography addiction, or to address neuro-motor cognitive skill deficits unthought of a decade ago (Pitts-Taylor 2016).

Back in the early 1980s when I took career steps beyond being a junior high school teacher to become a graduate-trained counsellor, I was captivated but torn by "the correct way" to understand and address clients' concerns. Early on, I recall reading psychoanalyst Theodor Reik's *Listening with the Third Ear* (1948), where each client utterance was linked to Freudian explanations that stretched any sense of plausibility (even Freud once said sometimes a cigar is just a cigar). I also read of the conversational wizardry of therapeutic greats like Milton Erickson and Virginia Satir, rendered by neurolinguistic programmers (Bandler and Grinder 1975) into scripted protocols to help clients make profound changes. I sought a science-backed way of talking with clients that I could use correctly and effectively. My graduate education then was also my first encounter with the kind of algorithmic thinking that often informs a medicalizing—diagnose and treat—discourse. This thinking was seductively certain, clients' concerns could be correctly understood and diagnosed, and properly treated with science-backed interventions.

Algorithms reduce complexities to actionable formulae (Steiner 2012) and require standardized understandings and practices (Bowker and Star 2000; Busch 2011) based on particular logics. Medicalization offers such a logic (Mol 2008) that has been translated into algorithms adaptable to counselling (Magnavita 2016) as well as self-care resources (Davies 2015). Protocols for obtaining salient information about client concerns, making sense of such information, and selecting interventions that should follow are consistent with the logic of a medicalized, algorithmic discourse (Magnavita 2016). In an era of EBP in counselling (Chwalisz 2003), such algorithms crystalize and operationalize protocols for a medicalizing discourse of practice, and extend the kind of seductive thinking I flirted with in grad school. Human concerns have correct diagnoses, and proper treatments to address them, goes the accompanying logic. The counselling approaches I later took up were modest and offered what one author referred to as "new languages of change" (Friedman 1993). They also addressed understanding and the constructive/deconstructive work of counselling as *discursive*.

Discourse/Discourses?

How do meaning and conversation—discourse—relate to what is understood, done, and accomplished in counselling? Answers to this question cue up strikingly different counselling approaches. Philosophers of language have also grappled with variations of this question. Charles Taylor (2016) recently cited two approaches to language use that have perplexed and polarized philosophers, and society in general. By one approach, language use *designates* meaning. Meaning of this kind is seen to have already been accepted and our uses of words are thus intended to reproduce established meaning. While our words cannot "mirror nature," to paraphrase Rorty (1979), designative meaning involves communicating through accepted and normal understandings that are often standardized as information, to be communicated and received as such. Language use that *constitutes* meaning has a different purpose, to make new human distinctions or "bething things" as Heidegger (1971: 151) once wrote. For reflecting team originator, Tom Andersen (1996), such uses of language are hardly innocent. While a designative approach sees language use as information exchanges for navigating experience, a constitutive approach sees language used pragmatically to negotiate experiential possibilities. For Taylor, the designative approach is monological (information transmissions/receptions) whereas the latter is dialogical (focused on negotiating preferred and effective, and sometimes new, understandings). Counselling straddles both approaches, navigating life by using established meanings while negotiating new meanings at other times.

Differences over Taylor's two forms of language use play a significant role in tensions arising from a medicalized discourse of counselling. The DSM-5 and the protocols of EBP are based on a designative, informational view of language use, such that human concerns have correct names (diagnoses) which standardized interventions can address. Professional conversation is the designative means to exchange needed information for diagnosing and treating medical disorders—premised on an "information transmission-reception" metaphor of communication (Lakoff and Johnson 1980). Turnbull (2003) similarly refers to a "code model" of communication involving information exchanges enabled by a presumptively shared logic that encodes/decodes messages sent and received. Precision in using established or standardized meanings when conversing is therefore paramount by this view.

Contrast this view of meaning and communication with a constitutive view of counselling, as dialogue without standardized or foundational meanings (Loewenthal 2011). By the constitutive view, what gets communicated is not easily translatable to pre-established meanings and protocols. People have conversational or discursive work to do, because language is used, or negotiated, for *purposes* that may not already be designated or preferred. Such negotiations have an element of linguistic improvisation between speakers by this constitutive view, as speakers "do things with words" (Austin 1962). They neither start from scratch, having to invent language; nor are their dialogues determined by established meanings. In Heidegger's (1971) sense, designative language is already there, its constructive use makes it constitutive. Meaning-making in this sense involves situated uses of language to satisfy speakers.

Considerable ambivalence can follow either designative or constitutive approaches to discourse. On the upside, designative language use enables people to communicate in presumed and established ways—we can learn to reason, understand, and communicate as others do, or are supposed to do. Relatedly, constitutive use enables new ways of articulating and imagining experiences—one person's depression may be otherwise understood as oppression, for example, for some counsellors (Wade 1997). On the downside, language can lose its ability to designate effectively over time; our terms can seem relics of previous cultural or institutional eras. A good example is derogatory terms used to describe learning disorders a century ago (moron, idiot). Returning to new constitutive uses of language, however, if these are not used in recognizable ways, they can seem eccentric at best; psychotic at worst. From a discursive perspective, what matters is what any use of language affords or constrains as possibilities (cf. Gibson 1979).

It can be the precision and standardization expected of people's language use that can be a source of tension associated with a medicalized discourse of counselling. Medical discourse exemplifies a designative and authoritative quest for certainty since so much can ride on its precise terms and professionals' uses of those terms. Spectacular advances in medical science (Dolnick 2012; Downing 2011) extended lives and improved many people's quality of life. Such scientific advances underscore the capacity of medical science to effectively identify diagnosable concerns and treat them. A rigorously practiced and scrutinized science can be used to adapt new technologies, test new theories, and evaluate interventions, and avoid the kind of quackery Ben Goldacre (2010, 2013) calls "bad science." Two human practices required for good science are representing and intervening; the former to identify, theorize, and classify phenomena while the latter involves manipulating and testing relations between phenomena (Hacking 1983). Thus, medical discourse has constitutive as well as designative uses, such as when new theories or diagnoses are developed (i.e. constituted). The poststructuralist (Spector and Kitsuse 1977) challenge to medicalizing discourse relates to the constitutive or designative values inherent in standardizing diagnoses, and to understandings left out of a potentially totalizing description.

Health itself has become an expansionary (constitutive) term and discourse, such that to the World Health Organization (WHO), health now means being more than being symptom-free (Smith et al. 2006). Being healthy has become a cultural project of targeting new aspects of life as diagnosable and treatable disorders (Conrad 2007). Human concerns or aspirations can be translated into diagnosable disorders, such as when Post-Traumatic Stress Disorder (PTSD) was added to the DSM-IV (Morris 2015); or former "disorders" like homosexuality were removed from the DSM-III. PTSD is a good example of medicalizing discourse having benefits; while the changes in DSM-III speak to changing cultural norms. Medicalizing discourse articulates and animates a particular logic and has enabled new ways of representing and intervening to address formerly non-medical concerns (Clarke et al. 2010) such as obesity or inhibited sexual desire. Medicalizing discourse focused on psychiatric concerns has amplified the number of diagnoses and treatments recently (Conrad 2007; Rapley et al. 2011).

Central to Peter Conrad's (2007) scholarship were "hyperactive" kids and adults who are now diagnosable and treatable for ADHD. ADHD exemplifies what a medical discourse's terms can afford and constrain. What is afforded by an ADHD diagnosis varies, but can include access to special education resources, pharmaceutical management of behaviors that might otherwise compromise the diagnosed person's capabilities and ways of relating, and understandings (self-understandings included) that recast the diagnosed person's behavior in non-moral (i.e. bad) terms. The constraints (e.g. being medicated) may not outweigh the benefits afforded by the diagnosis. ADHD also suggests a further understanding of medicalization that relates to minimizing or "governing" *chronic* conditions that cannot be cured, but instead can be managed with symptom-relieving medications.

The "ing" of medicaliz*ing* discourse relates to the processes associated with medicalization; in this book's case, as it pertains to counselling. Regardless of how well a medicalized discourse designatively accounts for a concern as diagnosable and treatable, there is inevitably something inadequate with its account. And so medicalizing discourse expands and modifies, constituting new meanings and practices needed to legitimize and extend what the discourse could explain. However, discourses, as we have discussed, can only partially account for any experience or phenomenon. ADHD is an example, and narrative therapists (Duvall and Beres 2011; Nylund 2000) seek conversations about what is unaccounted for in medicalizing discourse. Discourses develop or expand to address these unaccounted-for aspects, and for medicalizing discourse that means new diagnostic nuances, dissatisfactions with prior terms and discourses, and the development of new theories and research innovations. Medicalizing discourse has developed according to its own evolving terms, expectations, and logic. Counselling discourses develop to account for what medicalizing and other discourses leave out.

Medicalizing discourse also has come to legitimize what other discourses for understanding and addressing human concerns do not, given that it is developed through rigorously obtained scientific agreement on diagnosed conditions and the treatment or management of those conditions. This, for example, has been the view of advocates for evidence-based counselling (Chwalisz 2003). However, not all concerns brought to counsellors seem equally understandable or addressable in medicalizing discourse, or have even found consensus among health professionals (Frances 2013). The medicalizing discourse of DSM-5 and evidence-based treatments has stirred considerable professional controversy (Greenberg 2013), for what this medicalizing discourse's meanings and practice may unnecessarily totalize. For counsellors, expected use of medicalizing discourse can constrain other preferred discourses of practice when these discourses are perceived to lack scientific legitimacy (Strong et al. 2012).

Counselling and psychotherapy have seen their share of bizarre and dangerous approaches and interventions, and science has played a role in evaluating and sometimes discrediting them (e.g. Levant 2005). While antipathy between practitioners and researchers is frequent, discourse differences between social scientists persist over a "politics of evidence" (Denzin and Giardina 2008; Larner 2004; Walsh and Gillett 2011). Such differences often relate to approach-related or research methods-related disagreements on what counts as evidence in how human concerns are to be categorized. The disagreements extend to how research methods are used to obtain and discern evidence of change. Particular tensions arise for counsellors who are meaning-focused in their discourses of practice (e.g. Barnett and Madison 2012; Lock and Strong 2012), since client concerns are understood and addressed in fluid ways inconsistent with other discourses of practice, like Cognitive Behavioral Therapy (CBT), that use more standardized, medicalized discourse. The upshot of such discourse differences is that science has not resolved them with "gold standard" evaluations (Timmermans and Berg 2003), nor has professional consensus in counselling (Cooper and McLeod 2011; Duncan et al. 2010) aligned behind a medicalizing direction.

I walk a fine line here, I know. For readers who have already grappled with how science, language, technologies, events, and human interactions of any kind become interrelated (e.g. Barad 2007; Latour 2013) the kinds of issues I have been raising will not be newsworthy or controversial. Badiou (2007), for example, regards the "mathematizability" of discourse as important; with sadness being potentially mathematized through measures based on biochemical or psychological discourse. Two scientific and quantifiable discourses for the same event or experience—which one gets things right? Different discourses are common within scientific and professional communities (cf. Potter 1996), and tensions may come with standardizing terms, measures, or conversational practices associated with their use (e.g. Antaki 2004).

Standards, for Lawrence Busch (2011), are "recipes for reality," and when used in prescriptive or regulatory ways, counsellors sometimes push back (Postle 2007). Standards established through research also enable the development of different administrative resources, such as software and apps (Chun 2011), based on algorithms that reliably produce actionable judgments. Translated to counselling, such standards influence professional record-keeping, service rationing, and expected choice of interventions. This standardizing direction, though not transforming all counselling contexts, is a source of medicalizing tensions in counselling.

Medicalizing Discourse and Counselling

Standardizing counselling concerns under a common medicalizing discourse of practice may seem commonsensical for coordinated mental *health* services. However, counsellors have often approached clients' concerns through diverse approaches, developing and drawing from strikingly different counselling discourses to understand and address client concerns (e.g. Corsini and Wedding 2010). Social justice, existential, or relational discourses of practice suggest diverse ways for counsellors to engage clients. The assessment focus, the ways of assessing helpfulness, and even the role of the counsellor shifts dramatically depending on which discourse is drawn on for counselling (Paré 2013). While I doubt any counsellor would suggest that psychiatric symptoms are irrelevant to their preferred discourses of counselling, few would claim symptom diagnosis and treatment as the primary focus of their work either. Medicalizing discourse in counselling is based on diagnosing and treating psychiatric symptoms.

Where medicalizing tensions most frequently arise for counsellors is with justifying (Boltanski and Thévenot 2006) the work they do in the terms of medicalizing discourse, such as in administrative record-keeping, or in choosing approaches and interventions. In my research, some counsellors indicated that they infrequently experience such tensions since their payment or record-keeping procedures were not tied to use of diagnoses or related EBPs (e.g. Strong et al. 2012). Justifying, or accounting for one's practice solely on medical terms, tends not to be formally required of counsellors either. Some of the justifying arguably occurs in the court of public opinion, since people increasingly self-diagnose and self-identify using expert mental health understandings accessible to them through public media (Furedi 2004; Illouz 2008). Clients increasingly expect "treatment" based on a previously diagnosed concern, while needs to justify counselling on medicalizing terms seems to grow (Greenberg 2013).

Scientific (evidence-based) justification of clinical psychology practices hit full stride in the 1990s (Chambless and Hollon 1998), and drew from the methodologies of the Cochrane Collaboration on Evidence-Based Medicine (http://uk.cochrane.org/). The aim was to subject psychological interventions to the same level of evaluation expected of new pharmaceutical interventions. Some might ask where the professional dividing lines between clinical psychology, counselling psychology, and counselling are (or should be) drawn. Is counselling a junior sibling within the larger psychological family (Young and Lalande 2011), or is it even a psychological profession some might wonder. Such questions highlight how potentially conflated the conversational practices of counselling have become with evidence-based mental health and expected psychological interventions (cf. Busch 2012). Arguably, counselling remains a practice used by psychologists as well as other mental health and medical professionals. Part of the perceived conflation of roles like counsellor and mental health professional may come with how these terms are frequently used synonymously. Wikipedia uses the umbrella classification of *mental health professional* (Wikipedia, n.d.) to describe health-care or community professionals who improve mental health and treat mental illness. To the lay public, such distinctions may seem moot, counselling is less a professional title and more a service, albeit one usually offered at a mental health center. To counsellors, however, public or administrative fuzziness over how psychology and psychiatry relate to how they practice can be a source of medicalizing tensions.

Counselling as Researchable Psychological and Psychiatric (Mental Health) Discourse

Some of this fuzziness over roles and terminology is traceable to assumptions carried over from psychological and psychiatric research. First, the assumption that the concerns of counselling are reducible to diagnosable and treatable disorders *in* clients is problematic for many counsellors. Additionally, regarding interventions as "treatments" to produce symptom-reducing effects, as is common for pharmaceutical interventions, further reinforces this premise (Gabbay and le May 2011; Stiles and Shapiro 1989). The challenge for counsellors comes with how clients present their concerns. Are parent–child conflicts inherently about diagnosable and treatable disorders *in* the child, a family counsellor might ask? Is "trauma" or discouragement following a layoff a mental disorder? Does a husband's refusal to help out with childcare and household upkeep require one to diagnose the upset wife? To front-line counsellors, such discursive choices illustrate how clients' concerns can become translated into a psychiatric discourse that obscures or departs from clients' everyday understandings and circumstances.

A second, seldom questioned, assumption is that psychological knowledge and medical knowledge overlap, or even that psychological knowledge is foundational to counselling (De Vos 2012). As Boorse (1977) indicated years ago, health tends to be a normative concept and clinical psychology has embraced this view in ways that have concerned critical psychologists (e.g. Rose 1990). In other words, counselling based on psychological knowledge tends to focus on normal psychological functioning which, at first glance, seems appropriate. On second consideration, however, critical psychologists see potentials for counsellors to become instruments of dominant culture, perpetuating a normative status quo that may be unjust (Hoshamand 2001). A growing convergence of psychological and medical ways of research and practice as part of a broader, coordinated response to "mental health" spurred a current evidence-based movement in psychology promising professional legitimacy (Strong and Busch 2013).

In turning to the research on psychological interventions for particular diagnosed disorders, the most recurrent and significant identified influence on client improvement is the quality of the therapeutic relationship (Duncan et al. 2010). To those preferring conventional medical research and discourse, this is tantamount to saying that—across different medical interventions—a doctor's bedside manner is more effective than the medications or surgical procedures used. This could be seen as an argument for counselling, and less an indictment of psychological interventions for being modestly effective. Still, in an era when, to get paid or work in an institutional setting, for a counsellor to claim she or he is not using evidence-based interventions to treat clients' diagnosed disorders can seem unprofessional (Sexton 1999).

A final, theoretical assumption pertains to how intervention is conceptualized and researched as a component of the conversational work of counselling. Returning briefly to the communication metaphors discussed earlier in this chapter, it is the norm to see conversation as the means to do much of the work of counselling, to exchange information and give directives (Turnbull 2003). Thus, the conversational activities of assessment are understood as information exchanges, from which counsellors use assessment information to formulate a diagnosis and develop components of a treatment plan (cf. Seligman 2004). Therefore, interventions are seen as communicated by standardized prescriptions or psychoeducation through information exchanges clients are expected to take up to address their concerns. Unless improperly administered in non-standardized communications, interventions can be researched for their psychoactive effects, as in the example of research into the "dose effects" of psychological interventions (Shadish et al. 2000). Conversation in counselling is sometimes gauged by how effectively standardized interventions are administered to treat diagnosed disorders.

By a modern Newtonian logic of science, human concerns should be understood as engineering problems that have yet to find a correct solution (Toulmin 1990). In the social sciences, such a logic animates a current evidence-based approach to evaluating and prescribing psychological interventions, earlier adopted as legitimizing knowledge and practice in medicine (Goldacre 2010, 2013). While probably helpful in establishing standards of safe practice (Busch 2011) for counselling, evaluating counselling practices, as one might test medical procedures in randomized controlled studies, is where this logic can come up short. Human concerns are differently understood and responded to in counselling, depending on the discourses or approaches turned to. A medicalizing discourse of diagnosed DSM-5 mental disorders coupled with EBPs makes sense in medical contexts, but for counselling generally?

Pluralistic Discourses of Counselling?

Counselling is where different discourses in conversational use can be seen to critically and generatively interact as counsellors and clients talk together. Discursively oriented counsellors (i.e. those who focus on critically aware and resourceful uses of discourse) see their communications as more than information exchanges; rather, as reflexively contributing to relational processes they shape with clients through their meanings and ways of responding to each other (Gergen 2009; Shotter 2016). This focus on reflexive communications can make it difficult to distinguish what should count as an intervention, and suggests attention instead be turned away from specific strategies to possibly relevant nuances in the professional relationship. Thus, even questions have been depicted as reflexive *interventions* (Tomm 1988) for inviting new understandings and actionable possibilities. How clients and counsellors respond to each other shapes both process (conversation) and outcomes (meanings). For a discursively oriented counsellor, each person's opportunity for talking and listening offers reflexive possibilities to respond in ways consequential for the developing conversation with a client, while potentially identifying and amplifying client-preferred directions and meanings (Tomm 1988).

Two research approaches will inform how tensions arising from medicalizing discourse in counselling will be examined: situational analysis (SA) and institutional ethnography (IE). SA (Clarke 2005; Clarke et al. 2015) was developed in response to inadequacies Adele Clarke (2005) associated with classical grounded theory (Glaser and Strauss 1967). For Clarke, the inductive ("bottom up") qualitative approach of classical grounded theory produced tension-free accounts of complex situations, by seeking a unified thematic account that ignores the kinds of discursive differences we have been discussing. SA is a method for identifying and representing complexities and tensions in situations by distilling varied data sources into elements salient to situations, making it possible to map relationships between these elements. For example, funding for counselling might be one such element as might be a counsellor's approach to practice. In what ways might both elements be connected to and influenced by medicalizing discourse, the SA researcher might ask? Situations, like those where medicalizing tensions occur, are changing and contested, so part of the analysis focuses on where and how such contests are occurring. Conceptually, SA will inform how one might "zoom in and zoom out" (Nicolini 2013) of situations where medicalizing tensions are evident. Zooming out will occur when examining medicalizing tensions culturally and institutionally, by looking at the discourses in play. Zooming in will help to highlight instances where tensions influence clients and counsellors engaged in the conversational work of counselling.

A second research lens focuses on lived experiences and practices related to how dominance and resistance influence institutional and professional activities like counselling. IE (Smith 2005) is a feminist research approach that will inform reflections on the conversational work of counselling. IE offers an analytic lens useful in distinguishing between mandated or expected forms of institutional practice and the everyday practices of professionals engaged in front-line service delivery. Euphemistically, I came to think of this distinction as referring to the official and unofficial stories of practice, something brought home to me in supervising the doctoral research of Emily Doyle (2015), who contrasted such stories by speaking with staff in an addictions treatment center. Juxtaposing what institutionally is supposed to happen with what is experienced or done, is another way readers can relate their own experiences to those described here as medicalizing tensions in counselling.

It will be this zooming in and out, to consider how medicalizing discourse may shape macro and micro interactions of counselling, that will inform the reading ahead. Discourse will refer to the discourses of or approaches used in counselling interactions *and* the specific conversational work occurring within those interactions. To critical discourse analysts, and to institutional ethnographers, these systems of meanings are ideologies shaping important human interactions (Eagleton 1991; Smith 2005). Some may bristle at the word, ideology, being used to discuss medicalizing discourse, since it is derived from medical science. Thus, we will examine how medicalizing discourse was applied to aspects of life not formerly considered medical (Conrad 2007; Frances 2013), or to aspects of counselling where its individualistic diagnose-and-treat logic compels (or interpellates) (Althusser 1971) counsellor consideration. Medicalizing discourse influences not only externally observable interactions with clients and institutions, but also the "mental" reasoning (Wertsch 1998) or "inner dialogue" (Rober 1999) influencing how counsellors may (or do) clinically reason as they listen and respond to clients.

A common way to consider medicalizing tensions would be through social psychology's "cognitive dissonance" theory (Festinger 1957), where the focus is on cognitive consistency or disruptions to it. The purported consistency expected with cognitive dissonance theory is associated with the notion that personalities, and their understandings and actions, should stay consistent. Discourse theorists approach such tensions dialogically (Billig 1996; Wetherell and Potter 1992), turning away from personality attributes and toward differences over discourse positions (Harré and van Langenhove 1999) from which people might respond to each other as the source of their tensions. People can understand and act from more than one discourse position (i.e. they change "their mind"), so we needn't confuse personality with consistency of discourse use. Counsellors, for example, might listen or converse from more than a single discourse of practice to understand and respond to a client's grief over a recent tragedy, while resourcefully navigating and negotiating varied other discourse positions encountered when interacting with clients, agencies, and other professionals. Being aware of discourses and discourse positions can enable new forms of critical reflection and resourceful language use. In narrative therapy (White and Epston 1990) a common phrase is that the person is not the problem, that dominating stories (or discourses) can be linguistically identified, so that client-preferred alternatives can be considered.

Discourse analysts tend to look at such tensions in ways associated with identifying dominance of a discourse and how it is reproduced (Fairclough 1989) and through close examinations of what gets sequentially produced in people's conversational interactions (Peräkylä et al. 2008). Through such a discursive view social realities are produced in both macro-kinds (culturally or institutionally) and micro-kinds (dialogically or relationally) of interactions. It is in this sense that readers are invited to consider how medicalizing and other discourses vie for counsellors' and their own understandings and informed actions regarding human concerns.

Medicalizing tensions arise because other discourses of counselling can run counter to the diagnose-and-treat logic (cf. Mol 2008) associated with medicalizing choices. Very different clinical realities follow from these counselling discourses, though some are more reconcilable than others. In a proverbial free market of counselling discourses this would not be an issue, clients and fee-payers (not always the same) could choose freely. This is not, however, how the economics, administration, or institutional practice of counselling has developed. The tensions this book will address are those which arise out of expectations (institutional, public, collegial) that medicalizing discourse be central to the understandings and practices of counselling.

For Foucault (1972), discourses were hardly neutral ways of understanding and communicating, something evident when a discourse's dominance is contested. It is hard these days to practice as a counsellor without encountering the influence of medicalizing discourse, be that in clients' understandings of their concerns, expected uses of diagnoses when seeking professional reimbursement, or in justifying one's ways of practice as ethical. In Chap. 3 we turn our attention more specifically to how the human concerns brought to counsellors came to be increasingly legitimized through medicalizing discourse.

References

Abbott, A. (1988). *The system of professions: An essay on the division of expert labor*. Chicago: University of Chicago Press.

Althusser, L. (Ed.). (1971). *Lenin and philosophy and other essays*. New York: Monthly Review Press.

Andersen, T. (1996). Language is not innocent. In F. W. Kaslow (Ed.), *Handbook of relational diagnosis and dysfunctional family patterns* (pp. 119–125). Oxford: Wiley.

Anderson, H., & Goolishian, H. A. (1992). The client is the expert: A not-knowing approach to therapy. In S. McNamee & K. Gergen (Eds.), *Therapy as social construction* (pp. 25–39). Newbury Park, CA: Sage.

Antaki, C. (2004). Reading minds or dealing with interactional implications? *Theory and Psychology, 14*(5), 667–683.

Austin, J. L. (1962). *How to do things with words*. Cambridge, MA: Harvard University Press.

Badiou, A. (2007). *The century*. Oxford: Polity Press.

Bandler, R., & Grinder, J. (1975). *The structure of magic, Vol. 1: A book about language and therapy*. Palo Alto: Science and Behavior Books.

Barad, K. (2007). *Meeting the universe halfway: Quantum physics and the entanglement of matter and meaning*. Durham, NC: Duke University Press.

Barnett, L., & Madison, G. (2012). *Existential therapy: Legacy, vibrancy and dialogue*. New York: Routledge.
Billig, M. (1996). *Arguing and thinking: A rhetorical approach to social psychology*. Cambridge: Cambridge University Press.
Boltanski, L., & Thévenot, L. (2006). *On justification: Economies of worth*. Princeton: Princeton University Press.
Boorse, C. (1977). Health as a theoretical concept. *Philosophy of Science, 44*(4), 542–573.
Bowker, G. C., & Star, S. L. (2000). *Sorting things out: Classification and its consequences*. Cambridge, MA: MIT Press.
Busch, L. (2011). *Standards: Recipes for reality*. Cambridge, MA: MIT Press.
Busch, R. (2012). Problematizing social context in evidence-based therapy evaluation practice/governance. In A. Lock & T. Strong (Eds.), *Discursive perspectives in therapeutic practices* (pp. 245–268). Oxford: Oxford University Press.
Cecchin, G., Lane, G., & Ray, W. A. (1992). *Irreverence: A strategy for therapists' survival*. London: Karnac.
Chambless, D. L., & Hollon, S. D. (1998). Defining empirically supported therapies. *Journal of Consulting and Clinical Psychology, 66*(1), 7–18.
Chun, W. H. K. (2011). *Programmed visions: Software and memory*. Cambridge, MA: MIT Press.
Chwalisz, K. (2003). Evidence-based practice: A framework for twenty-first century scientist-practitioner training. *The Counseling Psychologist, 31*(5), 497–528.
Clarke, A. E. (2005). *Situational analysis: Grounded theory after the postmodern turn*. Thousand Oaks, CA: Sage.
Clarke, A. E., Mamo, L., Fosket, J. R., Fishman, J. R., & Shim, J. K. (Eds.). (2010). *Biomedicalization: Technoscience, health and illness in the US*. Durham, NC: Duke University Press.
Clarke, A. E., Friese, C., & Washburn, R. (Eds.). (2015). *Situational analysis in practice: Mapping research with grounded theory*. Walnut Creek, CA: Left Coast Press.
Conrad, P. (2007). *The medicalization of society*. Baltimore: Johns Hopkins University Press.
Cooper, M., & McLeod, J. (2011). *Pluralistic counselling and psychotherapy*. Thousand Oaks, CA: Sage.
Corsini, R. J., & Wedding, D. (2010). *Current psychotherapies* (9th ed.). Belmont, CA: Brooks/Cole.

Cushman, P. (1995). *Constructing the self, constructing America: A cultural history of psychotherapy*. Boston: Da Capo Press.
Danziger, K. (1997). *Naming the mind: How psychology found its language*. Thousand Oaks, CA: Sage.
Davies, W. (2015). *The happiness industry: How the government and big business sold us well-being*. London: Verso.
De Vos, J. (2012). *Psychologisation in times of globalisation*. London: Routledge.
Denzin, N. K., & Giardina, M. D. (2008). The elephant in the living room or advancing the conversation about the politics of evidence. In N. K. Denzin & M. D. Giardina (Eds.), *Qualitative inquiry and the politics of evidence* (pp. 9–51). Walnut Creek, CA: Left Coast Press.
Dolnick, E. (2012). *The clockwork universe: Isaac Newton, the royal society, and the birth of the modern world*. New York: HarperCollins.
Downing, R. (2011). *Biohealth: Beyond medicalization: Imposing health*. Eugene, OR: Pickwick.
Doyle, E. M. (2015). *'Recovery' in action: An institutional ethnography of addictions counselling work*. Doctoral dissertation. Accessed from http://hdl.handle.net/11023/2154.
Duncan, B. L., Miller, S. D., Wampold, B. E., & Hubble, M. A. (Eds.). (2010). *The heart and soul of change: Delivering what works in therapy* (2nd ed.). Washington: American Psychological Association.
Duvall, J., & Beres, L. (2011). *Innovations in narrative therapy: Connecting practice training and research*. New York: W.W. Norton.
Eagleton, T. (1991). *Ideology: An introduction*. New York: Verso.
Ehrenwald, J. (Ed.). (1991). *The history of psychotherapy*. Northvale, NJ: Jason Aronson.
Fairclough, N. (1989). *Language and power*. Harlow: Longman.
Fairclough, N. (1992). *Discourse and social change*. Cambridge: Polity Press.
Festinger, L. (1957). *A theory of cognitive dissonance*. Evanston, IL: Row Peterson.
Foucault, M. (1968). *Madness and civilization: A history of insanity in the age of reason* (R. Howard, Trans.). New York: Vintage.
Foucault, M. (1972). *The archaeology of knowledge and the discourse on language*. New York: Pantheon Books.
Frances, A. (2013). *Saving normal: An insider's revolt against out-of-control psychiatric diagnosis, DSM-5, big pharma, and the medicalization of ordinary life*. New York: William Morrow.
Friedman, S. (Ed.). (1993). *The new language of change: Constructive collaboration in psychotherapy*. New York: Guilford Press.

Furedi, F. (2004). *Therapy culture: Cultivating vulnerability in an uncertain age.* New York: Routledge.

Gabbay, J., & le May, A. (2011). *Practice-based evidence for healthcare: Clinical mindlines.* London: Routledge.

Gadamer, H. G. (1988). *Truth and method* (2nd Rev. ed.; J. Weinsheimer & D. G. Marshall, Trans.). London: Continuum.

Gergen, K. J. (2009). *An invitation to social construction* (2nd ed.). Thousand Oaks, CA: Sage.

Gibson, J. J. (1979). *The ecological approach to visual perception.* London: Lawrence Erlbaum Associates.

Glaser, B. G., & Strauss, A. L. (1967). *The discovery of grounded theory: Strategies for qualitative research.* Chicago: Aldine.

Goldacre, B. (2010). *Bad science: Quacks, hacks, and big pharma flacks.* New York: Farrar, Straus & Giroux.

Goldacre, B. (2013). *Bad pharma: How drug companies mislead doctors and harm patients.* New York: Farrar, Straus & Giroux.

Greenberg, G. (2013). *The book of woe: The DSM and the unmaking of psychiatry.* New York: Penguin.

Hacking, I. (1983). *Representing and intervening: Introductory topics in the philosophy of natural science.* Cambridge: Cambridge University Press.

Harré, R., & van Langenhove, L. (1999). *Positioning theory: Moral contexts of intentional action.* Oxford: Blackwell.

Heaton, J. M. (2014). *Wittgenstein and psychotherapy: From paradox to wonder.* London: Macmillan.

Heidegger, M. (1971). *Poetry, language, thought.* New York: Harper & Row.

Hoshamand, L. T. (2001). Psychotherapy as an instrument of culture. In B. D. Slife, R. N. Williams, & S. H. Barlow (Eds.), *Critical issues in psychotherapy: Translating new ideas into practice* (pp. 99–114). Thousand Oaks, CA: Sage.

House, R. (2004). *Therapy beyond modernity: Deconstructing and transcending profession-centred therapy.* London: Karnac.

Illouz, E. (2008). *Saving the modern soul: Therapy, emotions, and the culture of self-help.* Berkeley: University of California Press.

Kuhn, T. S. (1962). *The structure of scientific revolutions.* Chicago: University of Chicago Press.

Lakoff, G., & Johnson, M. (1980). *Metaphors we live by.* Chicago: University of Chicago Press.

Larner, G. (2004). Family therapy and the politics of evidence. *Journal of Family Therapy, 26*(1), 17–39.

Latour, B. (2013). *An inquiry into modes of existence: An anthropology of the moderns*. Cambridge, MA: Harvard University Press.

Levant, R. F. (2005). *Report of the 2005 presidential task force on evidence-based practice*. American Psychological Association. Accessed from https://www.apa.org/practice/resources/evidence/evidence-based-report.pdf.

Lock, A., & Strong, T. (Eds.). (2012). *Discursive perspectives in therapeutic practice*. New York: Oxford University Press.

Loewenthal, D. (2011). *Post-existentialism and the psychological therapies: Towards a therapy without foundations*. London: Karnac.

Magnavita, J. J. (2016). *Clinical decision making when the stakes are high*. Washington: American Psychological Association.

Miller, S. D., Duncan, B. L., & Hubble, M. A. (1997). *Escape from Babel: Toward a unifying language for psychotherapy practice*. New York: W.W. Norton.

Mills, C. (1940). Situated actions and vocabularies of motive. *American Sociological Review, 5*(6), 904–913.

Mol, A. (2008). *The logic of care: Health and the problem of patient choice*. London: Routledge.

Monk, G., & Gehart, D. R. (2003). Sociopolitical activist or conversational partner? Distinguishing the position of the therapist in narrative and collaborative therapies. *Family Process, 42*(1), 19–30.

Morris, D. J. (2015). *The evil hours: A biography of post-traumatic stress disorder*. New York: Houghton Mifflin Harcourt.

Nicolini, D. (2013). *Practice theory, work, and organization: An introduction*. Oxford: Oxford University Press.

Nylund, D. (2000). *Treating Huckleberry Finn: A new narrative approach with kids diagnosed ADD/ADHD*. San Francisco: Jossey-Bass.

Paré, D. (2013). *The practice of collaborative counseling and psychotherapy: Developing skills in culturally mindful helping*. Los Angeles: Sage.

Peräkylä, A., Antaki, C., Vehviläinen, S., & Leudar, I. (Eds.). (2008). *Conversation analysis and psychotherapy*. Cambridge: Cambridge University Press.

Pitts-Taylor, V. (2016). *The brain's body: Neuroscience and corporeal politics*. Durham, NC: Duke University Press.

Postle, D. (2007). *Regulating the psychological therapies: From taxonomy to taxidermy* (2nd ed.). Ross-on-Wye: PCCS Books.

Potter, J. (1996). *Representing reality*. Thousand Oaks, CA: Sage.

Proctor, G. (2002). *The dynamics of power in counselling and psychotherapy: Ethics, politics and practice*. Ross-on-Wye: PCCS Books.

Rapley, M., Moncrieff, J., & Dillon, J. (2011). *De-medicalizing misery: Psychiatry, psychology and the human condition*. New York: Macmillan.
Reik, T. (1948). *Listening with the third ear: The inner experience of a psychoanalyst*. New York: Farrar & Straus.
Rober, P. (1999). The therapist's inner conversation in family therapy practice: Some ideas about the self of the therapist, therapeutic impasse, and the process of reflection. *Family Process, 38*(2), 209–228.
Rorty, R. (1979). *Philosophy and the mirror of nature*. Princeton: Princeton University Press.
Rose, N. (1990). *Governing the soul: The shaping of the private self*. New York: Routledge.
Seligman, L. (2004). *Diagnosis and treatment planning in counseling* (3rd ed.). New York: Springer.
Sexton, T. L. (1999). *Evidence-based counseling: Implications for counseling practice, preparation, and professionalism*. Greensboro, NC: ERIC Clearinghouse on Counseling and Student Services.
Shadish, W. R., Navarro, A. M., Matt, G. E., & Phillips, G. (2000). The effects of psychological therapies under clinically representative conditions: A meta-analysis. *Psychological Bulletin, 126*, 512–529.
Shotter, J. (2016). *Speaking actually: Towards a new "Fluid" common-sense understanding of relational becomings*. Farnhill: Everything is Connected Press.
Smith, D. E. (2005). *Institutional ethnography: A sociology for people*. New York: Altamira Press.
Smith, B. J., Tang, K. C., & Nutbeam, D. (2006). WHO health promotion glossary: New terms. *Health Promotion International, 21*(4), 340–345.
Spector, M., & Kitsuse, J. I. (1977). *Constructing social problems*. Menlo Park: Cummings.
Steiner, C. (2012). *Automate this: How algorithms came to rule our world*. New York: Penguin.
Stiles, W. B., & Shapiro, D. A. (1989). Abuse of the drug metaphor in psychotherapy process-outcome research. *Clinical Psychology Review, 9*(4), 521–543.
Strong, T. (2002). Collaborative 'expertise' after the discursive turn. *Journal of Psychotherapy Integration, 12*(2), 218–232.
Strong, T., & Busch, R. (2013). DSM-5 and evidence-based family therapy? *Australian and New Zealand Journal of Family Therapy, 34*(2), 90–103.
Strong, T., Gaete, J., Sametband, I. N., French, J., & Eeson, J. (2012). Counsellors respond to the DSM-IV-TR. *Canadian Journal of Counselling and Psychotherapy, 46*(2), 85–106.

Taylor, C. (2016). *The language animal: The full shape of the human linguistic capacity*. Cambridge, MA: Harvard University Press.

Timmermans, S., & Berg, M. (2003). *The gold standard: The challenge of evidence-based medicine and standardization in health care*. Philadelphia: Temple University Press.

Tomm, K. (1988). Interventive interviewing: Part III. Intending to ask linear, circular, reflexive or strategic questions? *Family Process, 27,* 1–15.

Toulmin, S. (1990). *Cosmopolis: The hidden agenda of modernity*. Chicago: University of Chicago Press.

Turnbull, W. (2003). *Language in action: Psychological models of conversation*. New York: Psychology Press.

Wade, A. (1997). Small acts of living: Everyday resistance to violence and other forms of oppression. *Contemporary Family Therapy, 19*(1), 23–39.

Walsh, B., & Gillett, G. (2011). A post-structuralist view of evidence-based medicine (EBM): What EBM contributes to philosophy. *International Journal of Person Centered Medicine, 1*(2), 223–231.

Wertsch, J. V. (1998). *Mind as action*. Oxford: Oxford University Press.

Wetherell, M., & Potter, J. (1992). *Mapping the language of racism: Discourse and the legitimation of exploitation*. London: Harvester Wheatsheaf.

White, M., & Epston, D. (1990). *Narrative means to therapeutic ends*. New York: W.W. Norton.

Wittgenstein, L. (1953). *Philosophical investigations* (G. E. M. Anscombe, Trans.). Oxford: Basil Blackwell.

Young, R. A., & Lalande, V. (2011). Canadian counselling psychology: From defining moments to ways forward. *Canadian Psychology, 52,* 248–255.

3

Human Concerns as Diagnosable Mental Health Disorders

The labeling of mental disorder has evolved over time because the lens of cultural attention extracts figure from ground in many different ways.
(Frances 2013: 36)

How medicalizing discourse developed to have the kind of influence on counselling's pluralism one sees today has been a complex and very human endeavor. Evolutionary psychologists trace human psychology's journey through our primate predecessors (e.g. Buss 2004; Wright 1995). To even think and talk about thinking, talking, and feeling was a capacity humans had to cognitively grow into (Jaynes 1976). Historians of psychological discourse (Danziger 1997) and psychotherapy (Ehrenwald 1991) highlight, from the earliest records up to the present day, a recurring overlap of religious or moral discourse with forms of discourse known today as psychopathology, or psychiatric discourse. Michel Foucault's magisterial treatment of "madness" (2008) gets at one facet of what we will consider in our historical review of medicalizing discourse in counselling, but madness will be less the critical target here than conditions more commonly brought to counselling, like stress,

T. Strong, *Medicalizing Counselling*, Palgrave Studies in the Theory and History of Psychology, DOI 10.1007/978-3-319-56699-3_3

anxiety, depression, relational difficulties—concerns Greenberg (2013) euphemizes as human "woes."

Hermeneutic scholars (e.g. Messer et al. 1988) suggest that, while science may try to explain nature, it can only try to *understand* human nature. The understandings enabled through human discourse invariably offer partial understandings. How such understandings of human concerns found their way into contemporary medicalizing discourse will be our interest in this chapter, particularly how they became intertwined with the cultural preoccupations and aspirations of the day (Cushman 1995; Foucault 2008; Hacking 1999). Despite a common Darwinian narrative of science seeming to take us closer and closer to ultimate truth on human concerns, a different narrative emerges depending on cultural changes to language, circumstances, science, and morals. As Nietzsche ([1887] 1956: 188) rhetorically asked in concluding his first essay in *The Genealogy of Morals*: "What light does the science of linguistics, especially the study of etymology, throw on the evolution of moral ideas." Relatedly, the linguistic philosopher of mythology, Ernst Cassirer (1946) wrote of the "paronymia" (inherent ambiguities and distorting capacities) of human language when historically used to address concerns like those found in the DSM-5's classified disorders.

Undergirding the chapter's narrative is a poststructuralist and deconstructionist premise (see Derrida 1978) that efforts to linguistically name concerns are inescapably partial, and these sometimes obscure other namings to understand and address "those concerns." The journey to DSM-5 has been an arbitrary endeavor of pitting medical science's best linguistic constructions against what has culturally "mattered" (Hekman 2010)—ways of getting a linguistic handle on people's concerns of the day and circumstance. The next generation of practitioner-researchers is already at work on new nosologies and diagnostic distinctions, with more focus on neuroscience (e.g. Jackson 2016) or on how new diagnoses may enable counselling services to be covered by third-party payers (e.g. Wamboldt et al. 2015). This chapter aims to situate such medicalizing efforts in a historical and cultural context to account for how we got here. Central to the second half of this review will be a reflection on a largely Euro-American pre-DSM history

(Cushman 1995), and the five editions of the *Diagnostic and Statistical Manual of Mental Disorders* (APA 1952, 1968, 1980, 2000, 2013).

Some Historico-Cultural Considerations

Anthropologist Victor Turner (1974) described cultural responses to human concerns as entailing a process of moving from metaphor to calculus. In addressing a concern without a common description or name, there is often an initial search for apt metaphors—a kind of making "this" to be like *that* stage of linking the unfamiliar to the familiar. Unfamiliar and unwanted cultural experiences beg familiar understandings, and this is where mythology and language development have been most generative (cf. Cassirer 1946). Early philosophers and spiritual leaders persuasively tried to account for phenomena we now consider psychological and psychopathological (Danziger 1997). The understandings that found currency across diverse cultures and eras were those which crystallized the wisdom of the people implicated by them. For Ian Hacking (1999), such notions of human concern developed in particular "ecological niches," from cultural understandings informed by variable scientific rigors and explanations.

Foucault's history of madness (2008) chronicled how differently (yet normally for the historical context) "mental illness" was understood and addressed. To quote one of Foucault's mentors, George Canguilhem (1991: 226), "One does not scientifically dictate norms to life. But life is this polarized activity of debate with the environment, which feels normal or not depending on whether it feels that it is in a normative position or not." This shifting position on what is or isn't normal results in "moving targets" (Hacking 2007), mobilizing transient yet elaborate cultural responses—in variations of Turner's (1974) metaphor to calculus trajectory.

Debates have persisted since antiquity over what constitutes the humanly normal or pathological (Canguilhem 1991). Among scientists, the trajectory from guess to "fact" to discredited notion can be seen to have its arc (Fleck 1979). The concepts and language change: phrenology was once explanatory psychological language (Combe 1851), while addictions went from being moral problems to "diseases of the will" (Valverde 1998). More recently, phenomena like "Multiple Personality Disorder" (MPD) have arisen then disappeared from the psychiatric lexicon following critical scrutiny (see Hacking 1995), while new disorders associated, for example, with internet gaming, have shown up in the DSM-5 (APA 2013). Sociologists have often examined the language of psychopathology as a social means to address forms of cultural deviance (e.g. Illouz 2008; Scheff 1967). As humans, our fate is partly tied to what we construct and live by through our uses of language, an observation Vico put forward centuries ago ([1744] 2001). Even Western understandings of "objectivity" shift with time (Daston and Galison 2007).

Cross-culturally as well as historically, the psychopathologies of medicalized discourse also vary; and for conditions purportedly biological across humans (cf. Bracken 2002; Watters 2010). While anthropologists report common identifications of conditions considered psychotic, cultural responses to those conditions have been arbitrary (see Murphy 1976). One finds oscillating views in history and culture as to whether such concerns are best understood as moral or ethical deficits of character (Danziger 1997) or as evidence that one's biological constitution (e.g. the "humors") was suspect (Ehrenwald 1991). Indigenous cultures, worldwide, have enduring understandings of balance or concerns based on imbalance (e.g. Mehl-Madrona 2011). Locating human concerns inside the mind (for many, the brain) focused intense debate among physicians and philosophers (Makari 2015). These debates in turn focused contemporary cultural attention on healing practices to help in healing "the mind."

While books on optimizing emotional life have been around since antiquity (see Kingwell 2000), literary attention to emotional life grew in the early Enlightenment (Burton 1621; Smith 1759). A new historical view of humans possessing *selves* developed, associated with being autonomous agents with political and economic rights (MacPherson 1962). By the 1700s, early psychiatry began to emerge (Makari 2015), hitting its stride in the 1800s. For example, Benjamin Rush (1812), a signatory to the American Declaration of Independence and a "founder of American psychiatry," published *Medical Inquiries and Observations upon the Diseases of the Mind.* Early psychiatrists tended to take up roles in supervising psychiatric hospitals (Cushman 1995; Grob 1995) that were less treatment-focused than concentrated on ensuring housing and care for those considered chronically mentally ill. Versions of such "care" were epitomized by the institutional care provided at Bethlehem Royal Hospital, popularly known as "Bedlam" (Makari 2015). The diagnostics that saw people placed in mental institutions were imprecise, and it was common for paupers, criminals, and "sinners" to find their way into such institutionalized "care" (Foucault 2008). History shows a fine cultural dividing line between evil and madness. Someone could be considered a witch in one context and a crazy person in another (Torrey 1986). Phrenology stands out as an example of where presumptive cultural stereotypes of appearance, perceived as embodying psychiatric conditions, could become conflated with the racism or classism of the day (Combe 1851).

Intervening to treat psychiatric concerns also varied. Closer to the everyday upsets and stresses that are our focus, conversational interventions such as mesmerism were developed and evolved into what we now understand as hypnotherapy (Ehrenwald 1991; Hacking 1995). Therapeutic communications, in this sense, were seen to have curative effects; and later lectures by figures like Charcot featured hypnotic treatment of diagnosed patients, openly demonstrating new forms of expertise (Hacking 1995, 1999). Nervous conditions (e.g. Freud began as a neurologist) were seen to be particularly responsive to such forms of treatment, with conditions like neurasthenia common in the mid- to late nineteenth century (Shorter 1992). Shorter (2013) also historically traced what became of the once-familiar phenomenon known as the "nervous breakdown." For Shorter, people reported their emotional concerns using accepted or expected cultural, or legitimate, presentations of the day. Another forgotten disorder, neurasthenia, for Shorter (1992) seems to have "morphed" into what we now call chronic fatigue syndrome.

Hacking (2007) has described "looping effects" whereby expert language finds its way beyond profession-bound discourse, to legitimize everyday understandings and presentations of common concerns. Looping effects relate to an assertion by one of Foucault's mentors:

> It is impossible for the physician, starting from the accounts of sick men, to understand the experience lived by the sick man, for what sick men express in ordinary concepts is not directly their experience but their interpretation of an experience for which they have been deprived of adequate concepts. (Canguilhem 1991: 115)

The circularity implied by the term, "looping effects," relates to how people make sense of, then present their concerns in the expert idioms of their time and circumstance. This sociocultural view of discourse (Vygotsky 1988) sees people learning to talk and understand as do others around them. From earliest recorded history there has been a "self-help" element to expert knowledges that purportedly address people's concerns (Illouz 2008; Kingwell 2000; Starker 2002). Put another way, expert wisdom is crystallized into socially accessible knowledge and advice by which people come to "know" their concerns and what they can do about them. Such wisdom informs religious practices, such as those taken up by Christian Scientists (Cushman 1995), or moral crusades such as the temperance movement (Valverde 1998). So, while medical experts and philosophers were central to developing early expert helping discourses (some medical), such discourses came to also furnish different forms of common sense regarding human concerns and their amelioration (Foucault 2008; Illouz 2008).

Psychological to Psychiatric Discourses for Human Concerns

It took psychology's development as a social science to inform today's counselling discourses. While moral and medical discourses had been primary ways of understanding or explaining human concerns, concepts of an independent mind and psychology emerged from debates in political philosophy (Makari 2015). Phenomenological understandings were key to an evolving sense that human concerns could often best be understood as skin-encapsulated, mentally generated, corporeally felt phenomena (Richards 2010; Schnog 1997).

Psychology itself was home to highly variable metaphors for its subject matter (Soyland 1994) and that variability remains on full display in the concepts and discourses psychologists turn to today, to account for normal and abnormal functioning. Psychological historian Kurt Danziger (1997) suggested a "great transformation" occurred in the second half of the nineteenth century, a transformation of terms formerly considered part of moral discourse into those of psychological discourse. Taken-for-granted examples abound: motives, personality, emotions, and attitudes. That such terms have become part of the public lexicon exemplifies Hacking's (2007) looping effects, though many of the terms of today's medicalizing discourse associated with diagnoses and evidence-based treatments are becoming culturally ubiquitous (Jutel 2011).

Some critics refer to an "invention of the psychological" (Pfister and Schnog 1997), with Danziger (1997) finding an "already there" moral language for psychologists to name their constructs and human concerns. Such moral terms color what has been deemed culturally appropriate when considering emotional expression and social conduct. Morality has also been a culturally fickle discourse, and when translated to responsibility for modes of civil conduct it can be shown to fit hand-in-glove style with evolving notions of *individually* focused psychology (Prilleltensky 1994). Here is Norbert Elias (1994: 206), on civility and manners:

> Nothing is more characteristic of the unquestioning way in which even today, in thinking about human beings, the separate individual is taken as the starting point ... but always of the image of the single human being.

Psychological discourse foregrounds the individual as the origin of action and cognition, despite locating social or cultural processes and knowledge within individuals. There can be a chicken and egg thing here; to be subjects unto ourselves, we find that subjectivity informed and shaped by social influences. However, for Gregory Bateson (1980), significant implications follow such ways of "punctuating reality." Examples can be found in what it means to be "properly" schooled in emotional self-understanding and appropriate social conduct (Martin and McLellan 2013; Morawski 1997). Psychological discourse was central to supplying the needed vocabularies for such self-education projects; even up to our present-day vocabularies and measures for "emotional and social intelligence" (Goleman 2005, 2007).

For psychopathology to become part of medicalizing discourse, it first needed the individualizing logic of psychological discourse (De Vos 2012) to be embedded in a neutral and scientific language of psychology (Prilleltensky 1994). Though symptoms of schizophrenia were classifiable by the early twentieth century (Torrey 1986), the terms we associate with depression (Greenberg 2010; Horwitz and Wakefield 2007) and anxiety (Horwitz and Wakefield 2012) found new articulation in an emerging psychoanalytic discourse. Psychoanalytic discourse provided a unique means by which psychological and medical conceptualizations of human concerns could be brought together. In counselling's conversational work, the projects (i.e. human concerns) this discourse enabled were personality focused, and targeting residual deficiencies from one's earliest and closest relationships. While not as pervasive as a few decades ago, psychoanalytic discourse found its way into everyday understandings and conversations (see Freud's 1951 *Psychopathology of Everyday Life*).

It was phenomenological philosopher Karl Jaspers (1963; original first German edition 1913) who provided the initial comprehensive examination of psychopathology as it was subjectively experienced. To those subjective accounts, he developed an effective (over the tome's seven editions) linkage of existentialist philosophy to the different psychopathologies he described. This kind of descriptive and explanatory account contrasted radically with the "black box" thinking associated with behaviorist views of human concerns, concerns seen as contingent with external reinforcements (Watson 1925). Where Jasper's phenomenological approach to human concerns considered pathological focused inward to subjective experiences, behaviorists focused outward to mechanistic accounts of concerns.

This brief and selective history of psychological discourse prior to the DSM (APA 1952, 1968, 1980, 1987, 1994, 2000, 2013) highlights the varied ways humans have put language to concerns they want to address. The precursor to the first DSM was the American Psychiatric Association's (APA's) (1917) *Statistical Manual for the Use of Institutions for the Insane*, which was largely developed to register census data and comprised twenty-two diagnoses. The language associated with these diagnoses was primarily medical and biological (Conrad 2007), whereas discourses in counselling have focused on a broader range of concerns responsive to forms of human agency (Cushman 1995; Illich 1977). The expertise assumed to inform DSM development has accelerated its looping effects; with one recent critic bemoaning a growing "therapy culture" (Furedi 2004).

Beyond a psychiatric discourse to classify symptoms of psychosis, no discernible linear path or logic emerged to inform the first formal efforts at classifying human concerns into mental disorders. Instead, one finds distinctions that continue to prompt debate, such as whether there can be a dividing line between biological facts and social values (Wakefield 1992), or if a related line can be clinically drawn between the normal and the abnormal (Frances 2013). Such distinctions matter when considering the range of client concerns brought to counsellors, concerns which may not fit within a medicalizing discourse of symptoms and their treatment. It remains difficult to separate the moral dimension from the medical dimension of a presenting concern, as one can find evidence supporting both (Pitts-Taylor 2016).

Prior to the DSM-5's (APA 2013) publication, I used Fig. 3.1 to show the DSM revision process.

Some accuse the DSM's scientific committees of engaging in an expansionist discourse of deficit (Gergen 1990), and DSM-IV editor-in-chief, Allen Frances (2013) complained of "diagnostic exuberance." So, what does this thickening of the DSMs in Fig. 3.1 speak to?

DSM-I to DSM-5

In the normal classification activities of other scientists, refinements in objective classifications of phenomena are common, but so too are intense debates over what should or should not be included in such classification schemes (Daston and Galison 2007; Kuhn 1962). The

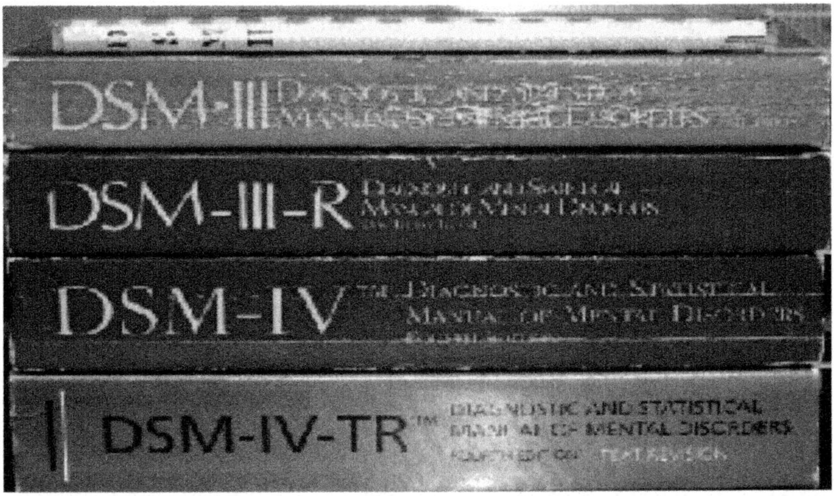

Fig. 3.1 Revisions to the DSM manuals 1968–2000

DSM-I arose from a need, following the Second World War, for a common language to enable psychiatrists to communicate about what they were seeing in the patients consulting them, and a desire to research the diagnosed disorders that had been classified. Therein lies a big tension associated with DSM's medicalizing discourse: researchers and practitioners contesting what is needed in a language of practice (e.g. Eriksen and Kress 2005). Recall, a key feature of any discourse is its inherent partiality; things get left out any discourse, and tensions related to discourse find their way into the conversations counsellors can have with clients.

It can be instructive to consider what prompted researchers and clinicians to identify and classify mental disorders in the first place. The first efforts were largely epidemiological and statistical, and aimed not so much at practitioners, but at census and policy makers wanting to better understand who was in psychiatric care and why (Grob 1985). While crude terms for what we now understand as mental disorders guided early efforts at psychiatric care (see Granville 1877), it took the world wars of the twentieth century to require a more refined vocabulary to align the intentions and understandings of researchers and clinicians. Agreement on what was meant by the term "mental disorder" was needed, so that it could be differentiated from the other linguistic constructions (e.g. moral/social deviance) that permeated cultural notions of "madness." Decades later, as these debates persisted, Wakefield (1992: 373) proposed, "disorder exists when the failure of a person's internal mechanisms to perform their functions as designed by nature impinges harmfully on the person's well-being as defined by social values and meanings." The word "internal" is key to orienting our medicalized consideration of human concerns, for this inwardly focuses attention based on a functional view of mental capacities, much like one might consider a functional view of mobility, vision, or digestion.

Mental disorders, as the APA (2013) presently states in the DSM-5, remain an evolving concept, but the continuing thread through previous DSM editions is that such disorders relate to disruptions to normal mental functioning. Normal is a key notion and reflected in the "S" ("Statistical") of DSM—with some of that sense of normalcy being related to a subjective view (self-perceived disruptions to one's normal mental functioning) and other aspects to how one can be sized up on society's presumed bell curve of mental functioning (Rose 1990). The concept of mental is also far from resolved, referring at times to behavior, cognitive functions, emotions purportedly regulated mentally, and so on. These things said, the DSM was developed to help *d*iagnose *s*tatistically significant *m*ental disorders *in* people.

In the early days, there was little overlap between the conversations of counsellors and those of psychiatrists (Cushman 1995). Counselling or psychotherapy was largely dominated by three approaches or "cultures" at the time of DSM-I: psychoanalytic, behavioral, and the newly emerging humanist-existentialist approach (Fancher 1995). As counselling discourses, strikingly different views of client concerns were formulated within each, yet only psychoanalytic notions of etiology seemed evident in DSM-I's primarily brain-based view of disorders. This conflation of mental with brain-based functioning solidified in the previous century but, historically speaking, this was not always the case (Makari 2015). It matters, however, when contemplating how conversation addresses human concerns as DSM-I diagnoses.

The 62 disorders (128 classifications) of the DSM-I (APA 1952) were delineated in 51 pages followed by appendices (the appendices start at p. 730 of the DSM-5). As the Foreword to the DSM-I indicates, three nomenclatures had developed (the prior statistical one mentioned, and one each from the US Army and Navy) translating to a "point of confusion" (p. vii) over the languages in use for diagnosing and discussing mental disorders. The DSM-I was developed to encompass and classify a range of brain-based disorders and mental deficiencies, through personality disorders and psychoneurotic disorders. It was the latter two classifications of disorders that showed the influence of psychoanalytic theorizing—something regarded as a problem for later editions of the DSM (Frances 2013; Grob 1991). The extent to which DSM-I came to influence clinical practice, beyond diagnosing psychosis, is little understood (see Blashfield et al. 2014), though its key influence was on helping to distinguish presumed organic from functional disorders. Its most enduring influence on counselling relates to the significance of psychoanalytically theorized personality disorders.

Those suffering from personality disorders provide a classic example of what Danziger (1997) refers to as "psychological kinds" of humans, language used to identify and classify people according to psychological traits. In medicalizing discourse, a personality disorder diagnosis suggests a major disorder to treat, if treatment is even possible. At his workshops on brief therapy, Bill O'Hanlon used to tell a story of being present at a case consultation where the counsellors would review their work in helping with different client concerns. At a few points in the consultation, the case manager would hold up two fingers, and the conversation about that particular client and concern would stop, and then the consultation would move on to the next client and concern. At coffee after the consultation, O'Hanlon asked what the two finger interjection was about. In the DSM language of the time, the two fingers referred to Axis II (personality disorders) and the case manager's gesture was to signal that this was not a client who could benefit from counselling. This example brings into stark contrast what classification can mean to counselling. Regardless, personality disorders continue to feature in DSM-5, despite major clashes over theory and related treatment in revisions up to the present DSM-5 (Clarkin et al. 2015).

While DSM-I helped initiate a standardizing direction for a diagnostic language of mental disorders, it also helped to further highlight tensions over what researchers and practitioners wanted included or excluded in the DSM-II. The WHO endorsed the consensual process used to develop the DSM-I, recognizing international confusion similar to that which prompted Americans to develop DSM-I. The Americans joined international efforts to harmonize their psychiatric language with one approximated in the *International Classification of Diseases (ICD)* (eighth edition), from which the Americans developed DSM-II (Blashfield et al. 2014)..

Early critics had mobilized a response to DSM-II's emerging psychiatric direction (e.g. Goffman 1961; Laing 1965; Szasz 1961), partly over concerns about human rights and dignity, though another objection was philosophical. Basically, however, psychiatry and counselling (such as the latter was), occupied very different spheres of practice. New to DSM-II (APA 1968) was a focus on concerns seen in outpatient services, not in psychiatric facilities. Specifically, though the psychoanalytic theory informing the presumed etiologies of many disorders was retained, greater attention was given to anxiety, depression, and childhood disorders than in DSM-I (Blashfield et al. 2014; Frances 2013). In other words, many of the kinds of human concerns—if understood on symptom terms—were classified and standardized in the DSM-II as counselling was moving into a very different era (Fancher 1995). Generally, early stages of "mental health" services were taking form, as changes to professions saw more counsellors join interdisciplinary colleagues as mental health professionals (Abbott 1988). Such interdisciplinarity brought its own tensions associated with harmonizing and administering counselling.

The period of the mid- to late 1960s was a very different cultural zeitgeist than the postwar era of the 1950s (Gitlin 1993). The human potential movement gripped the cultural imagination, as both counselling and psychology-informed self-help seemed to converge with a kind of spiritual or moral dimension focused on Maslow's (1968) "self-actualization" and Rogers' (1961) conditions and possibilities for optimizing personality development. It was an era the cultural critic Philip Rieff (1968) enshrined with a book title: *The Triumph of the Therapeutic.*

Later critics would come to see this era as fostering a belief in a potential perfectibility of humans under a term we now understand as "wellness" (Cederström and Spicer 2015). Counselling and self-help books were seen as resources for *growth* in this regard, and helped to usher in the 1970s as "the me decade" (Lasch 1979). While the DSM-II helped to bring a focus to less serious disorders, culturally speaking, a focus emerged on optimizing one's personality through practices associated with human growth. The final scene of the recent television series *Mad Men* showed character Don Draper having an epiphany (albeit a marketing one) after a long period of personal turmoil, at a growth center similar to the celebrated California retreat at Esalen.

DSM-II's psychoanalytic theoretical underpinning became a source of contention, perhaps best exemplified by debates pertaining to whether the eventual DSM-III replacement would include or exclude homosexuality as a mental disorder (Spitzer 1981). In the end, the issues were resolved with a vote, and psychoanalytic formulations of psychopathology disappeared and went into decline as well (Frances 2013). Psychopathology, however, was on the upswing, as the DSM II's 119 pages ballooned to 494 pages in the DSM-III (Blashfield et al. 2014). Part of the voluminous expansion related to criteria provided for making diagnoses, including differential diagnoses, while some related to a new politics accompanying discussions of what warranted a diagnosis, a politics one journalist covering challenges addressed by DSM-III editor, Robert Spitzer, described as requiring "nosological diplomacy" (Spiegel 2005).

The big change between DSM-II and DSM-III was a purportedly atheoretical shift away from psychoanalytically defined disorders to classification by diagnosable symptom clusters (Frances 2013). While the concerns articulated in DSM-III remained focused on disorders *in* people; etiologically speaking, these concerns became unmoored and a new kind of biologically oriented era of mental health emerged (Conrad 2007; Whitaker 2010). A multi-axial approach in DSM-III ostensibly enabled consideration of such things as symptom severity, life circumstances, personality, and other dimensions seen as helpful in making a diagnosis. Where counselling had been a resource to enhance human potential and overcome milder symptomatic concerns, a new form of pharmaceutical reasoning (Guze 1989; Lakoff 2005) was emerging, as psychiatrists moved away from conversational forms of therapy or counselling. Big Pharma had arrived while talk therapy, or counselling, was offered with or without medications as part of helping clients address their concerns (Angell 2011; Whitaker 2010). A diagnose and treat medicalizing discourse was becoming more common in counselling.

The DSM-III's (APA 1980) multi-axial diagnostic specificity enabled clinical research that later came to inform a revision, DSM-IIIR (APA 1987). Early adopters of this diagnosis-based clinical research were cognitive therapists (Blashfield et al. 2014), in a nascent evidence-based era borrowing from what had been developing in medicine to provide scientific support for use of medical interventions (Cochrane 1972). This diagnosis-based research direction, however, primarily came to be used to evaluate pharmaceutical interventions and establish ways to medicate a range of conditions that formerly had not been considered medical, such as ADHD (Conrad 2007) or deficits in sexual arousal (Clarke et al. 2010). While such medications had been developed and used since the 1950s to treat anxiety and depression (e.g. hear the Rolling Stones' famous "Mother's Little Helper"; Jagger and Richards 1966), prescriptions for new medications, such as Prozac, grew exponentially (Kirsch 2009), enough for one critic to refer to the increase as an "epidemic" (Whitaker 2010). DSM-III and DSM-IIIR amplified a medicalizing discourse of practice in ways that served administrative needs in mental health services as well, since the numerical coding of diagnoses could be computer-correlated with evidence-based interventions (Sharfstein 1987).

The DSM-III direction was also met with new criticisms informed by Foucault's (2003, 2008) historical and discourse-oriented writing, particularly with respect to psychology and psychiatry's roles in making "subjects" of people (Henriques et al. 1984). This critique came to focus on how cultural institutions *govern* normal as well as "pathological" forms of everyday life—in what Rose called the psy-complex (1979, 1990). A critical and hermeneutic turn also helped to interrogate some of psychology's most common understandings and approaches to helping (Gergen 1985; Sampson 1981). There were also growing feminist (Brown 1994) and cultural critiques of counselling practice, as a patriarchal and distinctly Western project for extending existing forms of domination. By the end of the 1980s, discursive approaches to counselling were also attracting increased attention among practitioners, partly based on a premise that counsellors could not be expertly objective in naming clients' concerns, that they had to instead collaborate through dialogue to find understandings and discourses that fit for clients (Anderson and Goolishian 1988; Hoffman 1990). Any dominant linguistic constructions of client concerns were seen as grist for deconstructive dialogues (e.g. White and Epston 1990) or as reasons to focus alternative strength- and preference-based dialogues (De Shazer 1985). In short, while the DSM-III added to the complexity, utility, and plausibility of a medicalizing discourse, critics saw what they thought was a last gasp of modern thinking about using language to understand human concerns correctly, in psychiatric terms.

If the DSM-III and DSM-IIIR amplified the number of biological disorders and diagnostic criteria, from what had been present in DSM-II, the amplification process escalated further with DSM-IV (APA 1994) and DSM-IV-TR (APA 2000). Robert Spitzer's protégé, Allen Frances, took the helm of the editing process, seeing the "DSM-IV, as a guidebook, not as a Bible, but a collection of temporarily useful diagnostic constructs, not a catalog of 'real diseases'" (Frances 2013: 73). This, as Frances realized later, was not how the pharmaceutical companies approached its use for specific conditions, as "advertising gold" (p. 73). The multi-axial dimensions for diagnosing mental disorders were further enhanced. Over 100 new diagnoses were added, as well as 300 pages of additional explanatory text (Blashfield et al. 2014). These "refinements" to DSM-III were developed within workgroups or committees and, as Paula Caplan's insider narrative on the personality disorders committee indicates (1991), the process did not always go smoothly, or scientifically. Caplan's concern was with a proposed personality disorder that seemed uniquely gender-bound ("self-defeating personality disorder") and so as a committee member she countered with another gender-bound disorder ("delusional dominating personality disorder"). Neither "disorder" found their way into DSM-IV.

It was also around this time that I first personally encountered clinical concerns associated with expected use of the then DSM-IIIR, shortly before the much anticipated DSM-IV. As a family counsellor beginning to use discursive approaches, I was working in a public mental health service in northern British Columbia. My specific challenge was with trying to bring a family systems and relational approach to assessment, to counselling families within a system that required DSM diagnoses (Strong 1993). In the family counselling I practiced then and now, the diagnostics, so to speak, were focused on relational patterns, and how to change them for the family as well as the family's "identified patient." However, clinical record-keeping and expected clinical judgments often required a medicalizing discourse based on diagnosing individual mental disorders, followed by treatment requiring use of EBPs. I was starting to see services managed according to how well these diagnostic and treatment practices were demonstrated and recorded (see also Wylie 1994).

The 1990s was also a decade in which the discursively focused therapies (narrative, solution-focused, and collaborative) were at the height of their popularity, with talk of a "new language of change" (Friedman 1993) or even a "Third Wave" (O'Hanlon 1994). What made these therapies discursive was the attention given to cultural and institutional discourses as they featured in the constructive or deconstructive conversations of counselling (see Lock and Strong 2012). In poststructuralist or discursive terms, the names or diagnoses for any client concerns were suspect; counselling was where new realities could be socially constructed with clients (McNamee and Gergen 1992). With these discursive approaches came greater attention to collaboration (i.e. power) and the ethics of such socially constructed counselling processes and outcomes (Weingarten 1991). For practitioners like me who were taking up these ideas, focus shifted to how to engage clients' expertise and agency, and for the counsellor that meant conversing within client preferences and resourcefulness (Anderson and Goolishian 1992). An expert- and deficit-oriented language (see Gergen 1991) focused on diagnosing and treating psychopathology seemed antithetical to how discursive practitioners should engage clients.

The medicalizing process toward developing DSM-5 became highly contentious. Criticism mounted over the extent to which psychiatric language was permeating Western culture at large (Furedi 2004; Illouz

2008), and non-Western cultures where medicalizing discourse was disruptive (Watters 2010). A league of critical psychiatrists, psychologists, and counsellors was growing, particularly in the UK (House 2004; Rapley et al. 2011), over concerns about expert relations configured by medicalizing discourse, and excessive use of pharmaceutical interventions. There had been a doubling down by clinical psychologists on expected use of EBP for concerns largely associated with DSM-diagnosed conditions (Chambless and Hollon 1998; Levant 2005; Roth and Fonagy 2005). This direction, too, encountered widespread dissent from counsellors who did not identify with the "medical model" approach associated with EBP (e.g. Elkins 2009). In the cultural mainstream, however, CBT's evidence base had prompted the economist, Lord Layard (2005), to prescribe CBT for addressing national concerns about depression, to counter the economic downside of a lack of "happiness." Depression hadn't usually warranted the same psychiatric attention given to psychotic concerns, but even at low severity it became targeted for medicalization, while also remaining a common concern brought to counsellors (see Greenberg 2010).

The anticipated arrival of DSM-5 catalyzed substantial resistance before its publication. Early on, the DSM-IV's Chair, Allen Frances (2013), raised concerns over its medicalizing direction. DSM-III's Chair, Robert Spitzer, had also gone public over the secrecy required for the development process, while professional organizations, such as the British Psychological Society, disavowed use of the DSM-5. Though a detailed review of specific changes brought by the DSM-5 is beyond our scope, efforts were made to further standardize psychiatric disorders in a more easily revisable language (this was why DSMIV's Roman numerals were replaced with Arabic numerals, to enable later decimalized refinements). A potentially "fatal" challenge came when the Director of the NIMH in America indicated that the NIMH would not fund research based on the DSM-5 diagnoses, preferring instead its own Research Domain Criteria related to neuroscience research (Insel 2013). This effectively rendered DSM-5 stillborn for research purposes when it was published a month later. While this position has few immediate implications for counselling practice, further revisions of

DSM-5 are to come with a planned, eventual, harmonization with the *(ICD)* (eleventh edition).

Coda

Returning to Wakefield's (1992) idealized dividing line between biological fact and social value, history shows that the line distinguishing a medically diagnosable mental disorder from unwanted aspects of the human condition (Arendt 1959) has been anything but clear. While psychotic conditions and brain injuries remain the disorders most would consider biological facts, in Wakefield's sense, other diagnosable disorders may be deemed as such because they counter societal values (Foucault 2008; Gillett 2009). In North America, it is not without reason that versions of the DSM have been referred to as the "Bible" of psychiatry (Cushman 1995; Greenberg 2013), but its influence doesn't stop with medicine or psychiatric practice.

References

Abbott, A. (1988). *The system of professions: An essay on the division of expert labor*. Chicago: University of Chicago Press.

Anderson, H., & Goolishian, H. A. (1988). Human systems as linguistic systems: Preliminary and evolving ideas about the implications for clinical theory. *Family Process, 27*(4), 371–393.

Anderson, H., & Goolishian, H. A. (1992). The client is the expert: A not-knowing approach to therapy. In S. McNamee & K. Gergen (Eds.), *Therapy as social construction* (pp. 25–39). Newbury Park, CA: Sage.

Angell, M. (2011, July 14). The illusions of psychiatry. *New York Review of Books*. Accessed November 17, 2016, from http://www.nybooks.com/articles/archives/2011/jul/14/illusions-of-psychiatry/?pagination=false.

APA (American Psychiatric Association). (1917). *Statistical manual for the use of institutions for the insane*. New York: National Committee for Mental Hygiene.

APA (American Psychiatric Association). (1952). *Diagnostic and statistical manual of mental disorders*. Washington: Author.

APA (American Psychiatric Association). (1968). *Diagnostic and statistical manual of mental disorders* (2nd ed.). Washington: Author.
APA (American Psychiatric Association). (1980). *Diagnostic and statistical manual of mental disorders* (3rd ed.). Washington: Author.
APA (American Psychiatric Association). (1987). *Diagnostic and statistical manual of mental disorders* (3rd ed., rev.). Washington: Author.
APA (American Psychiatric Association). (1994). *Diagnostic and statistical manual of mental disorders* (4th ed.). Washington: Author.
APA (American Psychiatric Association). (2000). *Diagnostic and statistical manual of mental disorders* (4th ed., text rev.). Washington: Author.
APA (American Psychiatric Association). (2013). *Diagnostic and statistical manual of mental disorders* (5th ed.). Washington: Author.
Arendt, H. (1959). *The human condition.* Garden City, NY: Doubleday Anchor.
Blashfield, R. K., Keeley, J. W., Flanagan, E. H., & Miles, S. R. (2014). The cycle of classification: DSM-I through DSM-5. *Annual Review of Clinical Psychology, 10,* 25–51.
Bracken, P. (2002). *Trauma: Culture, meaning and philosophy*. London: Whurr.
Brown, L. S. (1994). *Subversive dialogues: Theory in feminist therapy*. New York: Basic Books.
Burton, R. (1621). *Anatomy of melancholy*. New York: Wiley.
Buss, D. M. (2004). *Evolutionary psychology: The new science of the mind.* Boston: Pearson.
Canguilhem, G. (1991). *The normal and the pathological.* New York: Zone Books.
Caplan, P. J. (1991). How do they decide who is normal? The bizarre, but true, tale of the DSM process. *Canadian Psychology/Psychologie Canadienne, 32*(2), 162–170.
Cassirer, E. (1946). *Language and myth*. New York: Dover.
Cederström, C., & Spicer, A. (2015). *The wellness syndrome*. Cambridge: Polity Press.
Chambless, D. L., & Hollon, S. D. (1998). Defining empirically supported therapies. *Journal of Consulting and Clinical Psychology, 66*(1), 7–18.
Clarke, A. E., Mamo, L., Fosket, J. R., Fishman, J. R., & Shim, J. K. (Eds.). (2010). *Biomedicalization: Technoscience, health and illness in the US.* Durham, NC: Duke University Press.
Clarkin, J. F., Cain, N. M., & Livesley, W. J. (2015). The link between personality theory and psychological treatment: A shifting terrain. In

J. Huprich & K. Steven (Eds.), *Personality disorders: Toward theoretical and empirical integration in diagnosis and assessment* (pp. 413–433). Washington: American Psychological Association.
Cochrane, A. L. (1972). *Effectiveness and efficiency: Random reflections on health services*. London: The Royal Society of Medicine Press.
Combe, G. (1851). *A system of phrenology*. Boston: B.B. Mussey and Company.
Conrad, P. (2007). *The medicalization of society*. Baltimore: Johns Hopkins University Press.
Cushman, P. (1995). *Constructing the self, constructing America: A cultural history of psychotherapy*. Boston: Da Capo Press.
Danziger, K. (1997). *Naming the mind: How psychology found its language*. Thousand Oaks, CA: Sage.
Daston, L. J., & Galison, P. (2007). *Objectivity*. Brooklyn: Zone Books.
De Shazer, S. (1985). *Keys to solution in brief therapy*. New York: W.W. Norton.
De Vos, J. (2012). *Psychologisation in times of globalisation*. London: Routledge.
Derrida, J. (1978). *Writing and difference* (A. Bass, Trans.). Chicago: Chicago University Press.
Ehrenwald, J. (Ed.). (1991). *The history of psychotherapy*. Northvale, NJ: Jason Aronson.
Elias, N. (1994). *The civilizing process*. Oxford: Blackwell.
Elkins, D. N. (2009). The medical model in psychotherapy: Its limitations and failures. *Journal of Humanistic Psychology, 49*(1), 66–84.
Eriksen, K., & Kress, V. E. (2005). *Beyond the DSM story: Ethical quandaries, challenges, and best practices*. Thousand Oaks, CA: Sage.
Fancher, R. T. (1995). *Cultures of healing: Correcting the image of American mental health*. New York: W.H. Freeman.
Fleck, L. (1979). *Genesis and development of a scientific fact*. Chicago: University of Chicago Press.
Foucault, M. (2003). *Psychiatric power: Lectures at the Collège de France, 1973–1974*. New York: Picador.
Foucault, M. (2008). *History of madness*. New York: Routledge.
Frances, A. (2013). *Saving normal: An insider's revolt against out-of-control psychiatric diagnosis, DSM-5, big pharma, and the medicalization of ordinary life*. New York: William Morrow.
Freud, S. (1951). *Psychopathology of everyday life* (A. Brill, Trans.). New York: Mentor Books.
Friedman, S. (Ed.). (1993). *The new language of change: Constructive collaboration in psychotherapy*. New York: Guilford Press.

Furedi, F. (2004). *Therapy culture: Cultivating vulnerability in an uncertain age*. New York: Routledge.
Gergen, K. J. (1985). The social constructionist movement in modern psychology. *American Psychologist, 40*(3), 266–275.
Gergen, K. J. (1990). Therapeutic professions and the diffusion of deficit. *Journal of Mind and Behavior, 11*(3–4), 353–368.
Gergen, K. J. (1991). *The saturated self: Dilemmas of identity in contemporary life*. New York: Basic Books.
Gillett, G. (2009). *The mind and its discontents*. Oxford: Oxford University Press.
Gitlin, T. (1993). *The sixties: Days of hope, years of rage*. New York: Bantam.
Goffman, I. (1961). *Asylums: Essays on the social situation of mental patients and other inmates*. New York: Doubleday Anchor.
Goleman, D. (2005). *Emotional intelligence: Why it can matter more than IQ*. New York: Bantam Books.
Goleman, D. (2007). *Social intelligence: The new science of human relationships*. New York: Bantam Books.
Granville, J. M. (1877). *The care and cure of the insane*. London: Hardwicke & Bogue.
Greenberg, G. (2010). *Manufacturing depression: The secret history of a modern disease*. Toronto: Simon & Schuster.
Greenberg, G. (2013). *The book of woe: The DSM and the unmaking of psychiatry*. New York: Penguin.
Grob, G. N. (1985). The origins of American psychiatric epidemiology. *American Journal of Public Health, 75*(3), 229–236.
Grob, G. N. (1991). Origins of DSM-I: A study in appearance and reality. *American Journal of Psychiatry, 148*(4), 421–431.
Grob, G. N. (1995). *The mad among us: A history of the care of America's mentally ill*. New York: Free Press.
Guze, S. B. (1989). Biological psychiatry: Is there any other kind? *Psychological Medicine, 19*(2), 315–323.
Hacking, I. (1995). *Rewriting the soul: Multiple personality and the sciences of memory*. Princeton: Princeton University Press.
Hacking, I. (1999). *The social construction of what?* Cambridge, MA: Harvard University Press.
Hacking, I. (2007). Kinds of people: Moving targets. *Proceedings of the British Academy, 151*, 285–318.
Hekman, S. (2010). *The material of knowledge: Feminist disclosures*. Bloomington: Indiana University Press.

Henriques, J., Hollway, W., Urwin, C., Venn, C., & Walkerdine, V. (Eds.). (1984). *Changing the subject: Psychology, social regulation and subjectivity*. London: Methuen.

Hoffman, L. (1990). Constructing realities: An art of lenses. *Family Process, 29*(1), 1–12.

Horwitz, A. V., & Wakefield, J. C. (2007). *The loss of sadness: How psychiatry transformed normal sorrow into depressive disorder*. New York: Oxford University Press.

Horwitz, A. V., & Wakefield, J. C. (2012). *All we have to fear: Psychiatry's transformation of natural anxieties into medical disorders*. New York: Oxford University Press.

House, R. (2004). *Therapy beyond modernity: Deconstructing and transcending profession-centred therapy*. London: Karnac.

Illich, I. (1977). *Limits to medicine: Medical nemesis: The expropriation of health*. Harmondsworth: Penguin.

Illouz, E. (2008). *Saving the modern soul: Therapy, emotions, and the culture of self-help*. Berkeley: University of California Press.

Insel, T. (2013). Post by former NIMH director Thomas Insel: Transforming diagnosis. Accessed November 18, 2016, from https://www.nimh.nih.gov/about/directors/thomas-insel/blog/2013/transforming-diagnosis.shtml.

Jackson, P. R. (2016). The neuroscience of clinical psychiatry: The pathophysiology of behavior and mental illness. *Journal of the American Academy of Child and Adolescent Psychiatry, 55*(7), 632–633.

Jagger, M., & Richards, K. (1966). "Mother's Little Helper," song from the album *Aftermath*. Decca Records.

Jaspers, K. (1963). *General psychopathology* (J. Hoenig & M. W. Hamilton, Trans.). Manchester: Manchester University Press.

Jaynes, J. (1976). *The origin of consciousness in the break-down of the bicameral mind*. New York: Houghton Mifflin.

Jutel, A. G. (2011). *Putting a name to it: Diagnosis in contemporary society*. Baltimore: Johns Hopkins University Press.

Kingwell, M. (2000). *In pursuit of happiness: Better living from Plato to prozac*. New York: Crown.

Kirsch, I. (2009). *The emperor's new drugs: Exploding the antidepressant myth*. London: Bodley Head.

Kuhn, T. S. (1962). *The structure of scientific revolutions*. Chicago: University of Chicago Press.

Laing, R. D. (1965). *The divided self: An existential study in sanity and madness*. London: Pelican Books.

Lakoff, A. (2005). *Pharmaceutical reason: Knowledge and value in global psychiatry*. Cambridge: Cambridge University Press.
Lasch, C. (1979). *The culture of narcissism: American life in an age of diminishing expectations*. New York: W.W. Norton.
Layard, R. (2005). *Happiness: Lessons from a new science*. London: Penguin.
Levant, R. F. (2005). *Report of the 2005 presidential task force on evidence-based practice*. American Psychological Association. Accessed from https://www.apa.org/practice/resources/evidence/evidence-based-report.pdf.
Lock, A., & Strong, T. (Eds.). (2012). *Discursive perspectives in therapeutic practice*. New York: Oxford University Press.
Macpherson, C. B. (1962). *The political theory of possessive individualism*. Oxford: Oxford University Press.
Makari, G. (2015). *Soul machine: The invention of the modern mind*. New York: W.W. Norton.
Martin, J., & McLellan, A. (2013). *The education of selves: How psychology transformed students*. New York: Oxford University Press.
Maslow, A. H. (1968). *Toward a psychology of being* (2nd ed.). New York: Van Nostrand Reinhold.
McNamee, S., & Gergen, K. (Eds.). (1992). *Therapy as social construction*. Newbury Park, CA: Sage.
Mehl-Madrona, L. (2011). *Coyote medicine: Lessons from native American healing*. New York: Simon & Schuster.
Messer, S. B., Sass, L. A., & Woolfolk, R. L. (Eds.). (1988). *Hermeneutics and psychological theory: Interpretive perspectives on personality, psychotherapy, and psychopathology*. London: Rutgers University Press.
Morawski, J. G. (1997). Educating the emotions: Academic psychology, textbooks, and the psychology industry, 1890–1940. In J. Pfister & N. Schnog (Eds.), *Inventing the psychological: Toward a culture history of emotional life in America* (pp. 217–244). New Haven: Yale University Press.
Murphy, J. (1976). Psychiatric labeling in cross-cultural perspective. *Science, 191*(4231), 1019–1028.
Nietzsche, F. (1956). *The birth of tragedy and the genealogy of morals* (F. Golffing, Trans.). New York: Doubleday Anchor.
O'Hanlon, W. H. (1994, November/December). The third wave. *Family Therapy Networker*, 19–29.
Pfister, J., & Schnog, N. (Eds.). (1997). *Inventing the psychological: Toward a culture history of emotional life in America*. New Haven: Yale University Press.
Pitts-Taylor, V. (2016). *The brain's body: Neuroscience and corporeal politics*. Durham, NC: Duke University Press.

Prilleltensky, I. (1994). *The morals and politics of psychology: Psychological discourse and the status quo*. Albany: State University of New York Press.
Rapley, M., Moncrieff, J., & Dillon, J. (2011). *De-medicalizing misery: Psychiatry, psychology and the human condition*. New York: Palgrave Macmillan.
Richards, G. (2010). *Putting psychology in its place: Critical historical perspectives* (3rd ed.). New York: Routledge.
Rieff, P. (1968). *The triumph of the therapeutic: Uses of faith after freud*. Chicago: University of Chicago Press.
Rogers, C. (1961). *On becoming a person: A therapist's view of psychotherapy*. London: Constable.
Rose, N. (1979). The psychological complex: Mental measurement and social administration. *Ideology and Consciousness, 5*, 5–68.
Rose, N. (1990). *Governing the soul: The shaping of the private self*. New York: Routledge.
Roth, A., & Fonagy, P. (2005). *What works for whom?* New York: The Guilford Press.
Rush, B. (1812). *Medical inquiries and observations upon the diseases of the mind*. Philadelphia: Kimber & Richardson.
Sampson, E. E. (1981). Cognitive psychology as ideology. *American Psychologist, 36*(7), 730–743.
Scheff, T. J. (1967). *Mental illness and social processes*. New York: Harper & Row.
Schnog, N. (1997). On inventing the psychological. In J. Pfister & N. Schnog (Eds.), *Inventing the psychological: Towards a cultural history of emotional life in America* (pp. 3–16). New Haven: Yale University Press.
Sharfstein, S. S. (1987). Third-party payments, cost containment, and DSM-III. In G. L. Tischler (Ed.), *Diagnosis and classification in psychiatry: A critical appraisal of DSM-III* (pp. 530–538). New York: Cambridge University Press.
Shorter, E. (1992). *From paralysis to fatigue: A history of psychosomatic illness in the modern era*. New York: Free Press.
Shorter, E. (2013). *How everyone became depressed: The rise and fall of the nervous breakdown*. Oxford: Oxford University Press.
Smith, A. (1759). *The theory of moral sentiments*. Accessed from http://www.earlymoderntexts.com/assets/pdfs/smith1759.pdf.
Soyland, A. J. (1994). *Psychology as Metaphor*. New York: Sage.
Spiegel, A. (2005, January 3). The dictionary of disorder. *The New Yorker*. Accessed November 17, 2016, from http://www.newyorker.com/magazine/2005/01/03/the-dictionary-of-disorder.

Spitzer, R. L. (1981). The diagnostic status of homosexuality in DSM-III: A reformulation of the issues. *American Journal of Psychiatry, 138*(2), 210–215.

Starker, S. (2002). *Oracle at the supermarket: The American preoccupation with self-help books*. New Brunswick: Transaction Publishers.

Strong, T. (1993). DSM-IV and describing problems in family therapy. *Family Process, 32*, 249–253.

Szasz, T. (1961). *The myth of mental illness: Foundations of a theory of personal conduct*. New York: Hoeber-Harper.

Torrey, E. F. (1986). *Witchdoctors and psychiatrists: The common roots of psychotherapy and its future*. New York: Harper & Row.

Turner, V. W. (1974). *Dramas, fields, and metaphors: Symbolic action in human society*. Ithaca, NY: Cornell University Press.

Valverde, M. (1998). *Diseases of the will: Alcohol and the dilemmas of freedom*. Cambridge: Cambridge University Press.

Vico, G. (2001 [1744]). *The new science: Principles of the new science concerning the common nature of nations* (D. Marsh, Trans.). New York: Penguin Books.

Vygotsky, L. (1988). *Thought and language*. Cambridge, MA: The MIT Press.

Wakefield, J. C. (1992). The concept of mental disorder: On the boundary between biological facts and social values. *The American Psychologist, 47*(3), 373–388.

Wamboldt, M., Kaslow, N., & Reiss, D. (2015). Description of relational processes: Recent changes in DSM-5 and proposals for ICD-11. *Family Process, 54*(1), 6–16.

Watson, J. B. (1925). *Behaviorism*. New York: People's Institute.

Watters, E. (2010). *Crazy like us: The globalization of the American psyche*. New York: Free Press.

Weingarten, K. (1991). The discourses of intimacy: Adding a social constructionist and feminist view. *Family Process, 30*(3), 285–305.

Whitaker, R. (2010). *Anatomy of an epidemic: Magic bullets, psychiatric drugs and the astonishing rise of mental illness*. New York: Broadway Paperbacks.

White, M., & Epston, D. (1990). *Narrative means to therapeutic ends*. New York: W.W. Norton.

Wright, R. C. M. (1995). *The moral animal: Why we are, the way we are: The new science of evolutionary psychology*. New York: Vintage Books.

Wylie, M. S. (1994). Endangered species. *Family Therapy Networker, 18*(2), 20–33.

4

Legitimizing an Emergent Mental Health "Monoculture"?

A profession is always vulnerable to changes in the objective character of its central tasks.
(Abbott 1988: 39)

A relatively recent profession, counselling has developed in ways that outsiders might find confusing. While counselling's principal activity has remained clients and counsellors conversing about changes to clients' lives, the conversations defining counselling as a professional activity have varied considerably over the twentieth century. Similarly, counselling as a profession has undergone a variety of transformations that reflect these changing conversations. Counselling, however, has had to address some professional identity and scope of practice issues in response to regulatory developments, curricular changes in universities, "marketplace realities," and the politics of the professional members themselves. With the professionalization of counselling came competing requirements and claims pertaining to the profession's legitimacy in the public's eyes, to "neighboring" professions like psychology and psychiatry, and to administrators and third-party payers managing how counselling services are rationed. Terms like counsellor, psychotherapist,

T. Strong, *Medicalizing Counselling*, Palgrave Studies in the Theory and History of Psychology, DOI 10.1007/978-3-319-56699-3_4

and allied mental health professional seem to be used interchangeably these days—an innocuous development to the public, but less so for counsellors.

In this chapter I will historically reflect upon how counsellors have striven for professional legitimacy, and how medicalizing discourse has come to shape a continuing pursuit of legitimacy. It is a history interspliced with developments in social and medical science, but also a history of a profession responsive to societal needs and the workplace, showing how counsellors sought to make their professional services distinctive and legitimate. By what legitimacy or authority do counsellors engage clients in professional and paid-for conversations? Richard Sennett's comments on authority influence how I will proceed in this chapter: "In ordinary life, authority is not a thing. It is an interpretive process which seeks for itself the solidity of a thing" (Sennett 1981: 19). Counsellors seek to make differences in clients' lives on legitimate or authoritative bases that change with the science and circumstances of the day.

Counselling = Psychotherapy?

We should start by considering how the terms counselling and psychotherapy seemingly became interchangeable. Formally, the change in Canada is not yet a decade old as of 2017, and motivating the Canadian Counselling Association's (CCA) name change to the Canadian Counselling and Psychotherapy Association (CCPA) was a response to a similar name change to the British Association for Counselling and Psychotherapy (BACP). The reasoning behind the name change from CCA to CCPA was also decided by the Association's executive at the time, to position the membership for third-party payments by adopting the more prestigious term: psychotherapist (De Cicco, n.d.). CCPA was catching up with terms used in the professional literature for at least two generations (e.g. Rogers 1941; Truax and Carkhuff 1967).

Distinguishing between counselling and psychotherapy may seem trivial but the etymology of the term "therapy" in ancient Greece referred to *therapia* (healing) or *therapeuein* "to cure, treat medically," literally "attend, do service, take care of" (Online Etymology Dictionary, n.d.). Currently, the online Oxford English Dictionary (OED, n.d.) cites as its definition for psychotherapy: "The treatment of disorders of the mind or personality by psychological methods..." Conversely, the same dictionary shows the following meaning for counselling:

> [G]iving or taking of counsel; advising; ***spec.*** the giving of advice on personal, social, psychological, etc., problems as an occupation; in ***Psychol.***, a form of psychotherapy in which the counsellor adopts a permissive and supportive role in enabling a client to solve his or her own problems.

What do such etymological and dictionary distinctions have to do with how counsellors acquire legitimacy and authority as professionals today? In my view, they speak to trajectories that are sometimes distinguishable, but more often are conflated in the thinking and practices of professionals and the public who use their services, as the OED's definition of counselling suggests. These are discursive trajectories, referring to ways discourses develop to encompass historical developments and project into the future (Fairclough 1992; Foucault 2003).

While many forms of counselling are offered by other professionals and paraprofessionals (see Berman and Norton 1985), our attention in this chapter will be on counsellors who are registered by a professional association (e.g. CCPA or BACP) and hold at least a Master's degree. Counselling will refer to the conversational work of counsellors and clients that is inclusive of but not restricted to diagnosis and treatment of mental disorders. This latter definition is left open because counsellors inconsistently name the concerns clients bring to them, sometimes offering counselling with, but often without, the diagnosis of a mental disorder (House 2004; Proctor 2002). To the average citizen, however, counselling and psychotherapy remain interchangeable terms (Cushman 1995), and the same could be said for most counsellors who would similarly self-identify by both terms. Regardless, any review of the most common counsellor education textbooks today would reveal that the terms psychotherapy and counselling are both typically found in the titles (e.g. Corey 2016; Ivey et al. 2011).

The story of counsellors seeking legitimacy for their professional work is of course not restricted to appropriating more medically sounding professional titles. Psychotherapy largely developed in medical contexts with a focus on treating psychopathology, and with Freud being considered its modern founder (Cushman 1995; Ehrenwald 1991). Counselling in North America developed as a profession partly in response to the needs of the job market, and in its early stages was associated with the educational and vocational guidance movement in schools (Davis 1914; Hartung and Blustein 2002; Proctor et al. 1931). In a prescient article from the early 1980s, Aubrey (1983) described counselling as largely atheoretical, having a focus on helping young people to adjust to tumultuous societal and economic changes. The "guidance" focus of early counselling was enhanced by the relational and communications focus Rogers (1941) brought through his person-centered approach. This focus was evident in the primary counselling journal in the profession's early day: the *Personnel and Guidance Journal* of the American Personnel and Guidance Association. What made Aubrey's article prescient, however, was his 1983 concern that counselling was becoming divided over how medical its focus was to be, as it was turning away from addressing social concerns through problem-solving and decision-making assistance associated with the profession's roots in service as he saw them:

> The major concern with the counseling profession at the present time is its lack of focus and attention. One resolve is to establish work with youth and emerging social issues as the major focus of the coming decades. This would be followed by setting priorities for these issues, creation of appropriate intervention strategies, and the getting on with the business of helping people before disaster strikes. After all, this is really how the counseling profession began, and it wasn't a bad beginning! (Aubrey 1983: 82)

Aubrey was lamenting a more medically oriented counselling or psychotherapy. "Guidance," for many, was not only a concept for schools and young people, it spoke to the origins of family counselling as well, though focused on addressing problems "in" children, and (more often) to enhance relationships parents had with their children (Nichols and

Schwartz 2008). The guidance and counselling services in schools and at the child guidance centers of the 1920s and 1930s contrasted with the primarily psychoanalytically oriented psychiatric clinics and university clinics for psychotherapy services (VandenBos et al. 1992).

Counselling's Commingling with Academic Psychology

While counselling's early days primarily focused on addressing the educational, developmental, and vocational needs of young people, academic psychologists were taking psychology out of labs and into everyday applications where boundary-blurring was occurring between counselling and psychotherapy. While such boundaries were never clear or intentional in the early days of counselling—that came later as professional counselling associations emerged—psychological science would take on an increasing role in informing and evaluating new theories and practices used in counselling. Carl Rogers' (1941) contributions were a welcome response to the sterile behaviorist, and somewhat mysticized and personality-focused psychoanalytic psychotherapy orientations of the day. Skepticism grew toward a prescribed and objective detachment by counsellor or psychologist in diagnosing and treating client concerns. Counselling, in these middle years (Leahy et al. 2015) would take on a more humanized direction focused on the quality of communicating and relating occurring between counsellor and clients. It was also a time when systematic approaches to counselling and "guidance" were developed and advocated (Mathewson 1949). As VandenBos et al. (1992: 76) indicated, the Second World War was an era which:

> forced a broadening in the conceptualization of mental health ideology and treatment from the exclusive reliance on personal pathology to an expansion in the thinking and activities of mental health professionals, particularly among those with interests in psychotherapy.

Counselling in North America found its theoretical and research footing in university counselling centers that served as testing grounds for future approaches to practice. The early approaches to counselling were found wanting by psychologists working in such settings, so they pushed for more scientific and systematic approaches (e.g. Murray 1938). Psychology's eventual answer to this concern was the Boulder model, which was developed to bring together the skills of clinical research with those of clinical practice under a scientist-practitioner approach to practice (Frank 1984). In a more recent review of the Boulder model's influence on *counselling psychology*, Myers (2007: 795) described ongoing tensions between science and practice, and a prescriptive stance, as practitioners "are ethically bound to provide the most efficient and effective *treatments* available" (emphasis added). Such prescriptions create medicalizing tensions for counsellors at odds with standardizing how to diagnose and "treat" client concerns.

Where counsellors had previously been more focused on assisting clients with problems and difficulties, clinical psychologists tended to join psychiatric colleagues and focus on the treatable mental illnesses and personality disorders of clients. One common distinction between clinical psychologists and counselling psychologists has been over the primary focus each has on diagnosing and treating mental disorders with EBPs—something clinical psychologists purportedly do more of, by treating disorders of greater symptomatic severity than do counselling psychologists (Ogunfowora and Drapeau 2008). By such gauges of severity, counsellors are even further down the symptom-focused professional ladder since they focus less on a disease model of mental disorders and more on helping clients overcome concerns, while doing preventive and developmental work (Gazzola and Smith 2007). Still, tensions persist over furthering this medicalizing direction within counselling psychology (Chwalisz 2003; Hage 2003; Young and Lalande 2011) and counselling (Eriksen and Kress 2006; Pearce 2014).

An Emerging Mental Health Era

The aftermath of the Second World War made it evident that addressing people's "mental health" needs adequately required the efforts of more than just psychiatrists (VandenBos et al. 1992). The United States government sought to better understand these mental health needs by enlisting the APA and American Medical Association to oversee research for the Joint Commission on Mental Illness and Health (*New England Journal of Medicine* 1956). In reviewing the findings and recommendations of this massive and highly influential undertaking (which was published in six volumes), Cumming (1962) was highly critical of one of the primary recommendations: that mental health be shifted out of the large psychiatric hospitalities and into community-based facilities, then understaffed by mental health professionals (not just psychiatrists). The subsequent answer to the concern Cumming and others raised was substantially increased funding of community-based mental health services, and with that expansion of services, the training of mental health professionals, counsellors included, became a priority.

The 1960s were in a sense a large-scale social experiment where counsellors in a new era of community-based mental health had a significant role to play. In the years prior to the Joint Commission on Mental Illness and Health recommendations, counsellors increasingly came to organize as professional associations, as exemplified by the eventual emergence of the American Personnel and Guidance Association in 1952 (known as the American Counseling Association (ACA) after 1992; see Aubrey 1977). Similar organizations developed much later in Canada (the Canadian Guidance and Counselling Association, 1965, now the CCPA), and in the United Kingdom BAC (1977). However, it is within the professional associations, particularly their journals, that one finds the great debates taking place over how counselling would evolve (e.g. Aubrey 1983). The professional associations played increasing roles in articulating, legitimizing, and forging the professional identities and profession-sanctioned practices of counsellors (e.g. Gazzola and Smith 2007). By extension, such professional identity-shaping debates found their counterparts in graduate counsellor education programs from which they drew their academic advocates.

The university played a central role in both developing and legitimizing the profession of counselling, and in counselling's early years this was a wide-ranging challenge. The profession's intellectual and professional direction developed primarily through the leadership of academics in such profession-defining activities as articulating core competencies (e.g. Jevne 1981), developing professional standards and ethics (e.g. CCA 1989), developing theoretical models (e.g. Havighurst 1952), evaluating new counselling interventions (e.g. Hoffnung 1969; Shlien and Zimring 1966), and authoring the standard textbooks for the profession (Carkhuff 1972; Wrenn 1962). The sense to convey here is of the centrality of universities and professors in activities related to legitimizing professional counselling, to an expectant public (i.e. government). These professors were also central to a further development in the legitimizing process: establishing accreditation standards and procedures for counsellor education programs (e.g. Peavy et al. 1982; Robertson and Borgen 2016).

The thread that historically links such university-centric contributions to the influence of medicalizing discourse on counselling may seem obscure. Developing and legitimizing counselling through such contributions has parallels in other professions that counsellors have sometimes emulated, such as clinical psychology and psychiatry. In this respect, counselling could be seen to have progressed by drawing on profession-legitimizing practices common to more established and prestigious professions. In so doing, counselling developed in ways consistent with Abbott's (1988: 56–57) analysis: "the academic knowledge system of a profession generally accomplishes three tasks—legitimation, research, and instruction—and in each it shapes the vulnerability of professional jurisdiction to outside interference." My aim is to show recursive and reinforcing links between these tasks, in efforts to legitimize a relatively young profession. A more elusive challenge is to show how medicalization afforded a new and compelling means to legitimize counselling through research and professional education.

The era in which counselling became commonplace—through enhanced funding, new professional organizations, its first textbooks, and so on—was also the era in which science was putting astronauts in space and eradicating diseases like polio. Scientists were to play a central role in an increasingly technocratic society where their pursuit of knowledge was considered heroic and virtuous (Shapin 2008). While social science lagged behind medical science and aeronautical engineering, for many it seemed an inevitability that the science of psychology, in tandem with developments in psychiatry, would eventually deliver a much enhanced quality of life to society at large. Counselling and psychology were pulled in this technocratic direction (e.g. Skinner 1972), while, in another direction, the ceiling seemed off what counselling and psychological knowledge offered human potential (e.g. Maslow 1971; Perls 1969). Counselling was in an expansionary phase and with that came some excesses and cautionary tales.

Richard Sennett (1981) suggested that legitimate personal authority is perceived to relate to one's ability to judge and reassure others on the basis of respected knowledge. Translated to a counsellor's legitimate authority, what were these abilities to judge and reassure? Answers to this question varied widely, particularly in the 1960s and 1970s. Counselling entered a new phase of popular existentialist, social justice, and humanist ideas and practices (Schutz 1967; see the evolution described in Ferguson 1980, and criticized by Rosen 1978). This transformation was occurring at the same time as behavioral psychology offered promising understandings for socially engineering modifications in human behavior (e.g. Bandura 1969; Wolpe 1958). It was also a time when abuses of institutional psychiatry were publicly recounted (Goffman 1961; Kesey 1962). Finally, a large-scale transition from hospitals and expensive private practices, into community mental health centers for the public occurred. For counsellors, being recognized as a legitimate source of help could mean many things given these cultural developments.

With counsellors' (i.e. mental health) services being made more publicly accessible, more trained counsellors were needed to take up roles in community schools, mental health centers, and other outreach services in order to help a growing clientele. Most of these new counsellors were graduates of counsellor education Master's programs, for an occupation that was upscaling itself to become a profession (see Leahy et al. 2015). The curriculum of the 1970s and 1980s tended to be a grab bag of theoretical approaches that prompted some academics to develop unifying systems while others sought to remain eclectic, or deliberately specialized (Aubrey 1977). Research evaluating specialized counselling approaches (e.g. Gestalt) for their effectiveness, or their unification, was in its infancy. Carl Rogers' conversational practices, however, had been transformed into teachable, researchable counsellor micro-skills central to graduate counsellor education (e.g. Carkhuff 1969). Early counselling research focused on career interventions (Holland et al. 1981) or measuring aspects of the counselling relationship (e.g. Bordin 1979). Apart from such research, counsellor education in the 1970s tended to focus on counselling micro-skills and largely untested theoretical approaches and interventions.

The 1970s also became referred to as the "me decade" (Ringer 1977; Sampson 1977) for a number of reasons, but most relevant to our context was a publicly growing, yet subjective, focus on personal development and assertiveness (Alberti and Emmons 1970; Boston Women's Health Collective 1971). Counselling had become a resource for empowerment, influenced in part by a self-help literature that came to be known as "pop psychology," and that amplified circulation of 1960s-era human potential ideas. This literature also circulated details for previously unrecognized psychological concerns, providing prospective counselling clients with new bases for self-diagnosing (see Furedi 2004; Hacking 1995; Illouz 2008). As counselling services expanded, distinctions between counselling based on medicalizing discourse (i.e. diagnosing and treating mental disorders) and counselling for other human concerns (Aubrey's problems and difficulties, Aubrey 1983) grew less clear.

DSM-III and Legitimizing Counselling

The arrival of DSM-III in 1980 was to provide a transformative and unifying language for mental health practitioners (Wilson 1993); it was also a "cultural phenomenon" (Spiegel 2005). What the DSM-III did accomplish was identify many more diagnosable symptom clusters, accelerating the number of disorders considered primarily biomedical in nature. This acceleration greatly influenced research and later research-informed developments that would have a major bearing on the practice of counselling in non-psychiatric contexts. The language of DSM provided a conceptual and unifying framework from which research of mental health practice could begin. While largely focused on measuring the effectiveness of medications for treating diagnosed mental disorders (see Whitaker 2010), such research was also helpful in conceptualizing and evaluating psychotherapeutic interventions. EBP, as it was then known in counselling, would not have been possible without the standardization of mental health practices and knowledge for diagnosing and treating "mental disorders" considered primarily biomedical in nature (Busch 2011; Timmermans and Berg 2003).

It is important to unpack what this standardizing means when it comes to linking such research to its practical applications. The primary aim of standardization is to reduce naturally occurring variability through establishing conditions or procedures leading to outcomes that can be reliably reproduced (Busch 2011; Timmermans and Berg 2003). Put paradigmatically, the conditions and procedures used in highly controlled experimental evaluations are to be replicated in actual situations of clinical practice, like counselling. This, of course, is an idealization (or distortion) of what might transpire in the actual conversations between client and counsellor. It also relates to a concern Foucault (1978) had about professionals needing "docile bodies" to accomplish their work. Despite what the research literature sometimes indicates, counsellors don't administer "doses" of interventions to clients as one might administer a medication (Stiles and Shapiro 1989). There's a "responsiveness" issue by participants (clients) that even the best interventions researchers can't control for procedurally or statistically (Kramer and Stiles 2015). To conversationally administer such interventions, clients misunderstood, disagree, hear in their own ways, and so on—uncontrollable factors contributing to this research responsiveness issue. Counsellors obviously don't have docile clients, and their conversations entail more than exchanges of information or administrations of conversationally oriented interventions that researchers have deemed effective under highly controlled conditions.

Even in efforts to standardize diagnostic procedures so that the diagnosed conditions being researched or "treated" are considered reliably and validly diagnosed, one finds considerable variability (Kutchins and Kirk 2003). Variability is the antithesis of standardized practice and invites a kind of professional scorn, particularly from practitioner-researchers invested in ensuring that practice is done "right" (Timmermans and Berg 2003; Tucker and Blythe 2008).

For administrators expecting such fidelity from clinicians in following diagnostic and treatment procedures, variability is a major systems and quality control issue (Tanenbaum 2013). To properly administer services, in what Rose (1979) long ago referred to as the psy-complex, one needs algorithms that can ensure services are delivered based on proper adherence to diagnostic and treatment protocols (see Downing 2011; Steiner 2012).

What the psychiatric research based on the DSM-III enabled were new administrative guidelines, or protocols for diagnosing (e.g. Jensen et al. 1995) and treating mental disorders (e.g. Wessler and Hankin-Wessler 1989). While such evidence-informed developments did not initially target counsellors specifically, the mental health services where they worked increasingly took up this approach to practice. Advocacy eventually developed within psychology (Chambless and Hollon 1998) and counselling (Chwalisz 2003) to move in this direction. An evidence-based approach, suggest Cartwright and Hardie (2012: 42), requires belief in the transferability of what is produced in experimental conditions:

> [T]hat "it works there" gives information about the causal principle that obtains there and about the existence of the requisite support factors there. But it gives no information about what the causal principle here is nor about what support factors, if any, obtain here.

This transferability relates to the generalizability claims of social scientists, for whom "there" and "here," as the quote suggests, should proceed and be subject to the same causal principles. Generalizability requires standardizing practice, or ensuring "treatment fidelity" (Borrelli et al. 2005). Treatment fidelity is a standardizing logic and expectation that translates well to administrative requirements. By a similar logic; such standardizing efforts get one a similar McDonald's © hamburger in Seattle and Stockholm. Regardless of the practice setting, administrative decisions could similarly be based on reliably adhered to diagnostic protocols, followed by treatment using standardized intervention protocols for the diagnosed disorder. This might seem an excessive characterization irrelevant to the immediacies of counselling, but it is a kind of quintessentially modern managerialism or bureaucratization, and a source of concern for some counsellors (House 2004; Pearce 2014; Postle 2007).

EBP, primarily the approach imported from medicine (http://www.cochrane.org/), has been central to the push from within the American Psychological Association's Clinical Psychology Division (Chambless and Hollon 1998) to legitimize the knowledge and practices of psychologists. Where DSM-III had enabled a first step in a profession-wide research program for restoring legitimacy to psychiatry (Frances 2013), like other evidence-based research in medicine it had the double-edged mandate of ensuring safe medical interventions and evaluating safe interventions for their effectiveness. Clinical psychologists were playing catch up with what had been happening through the Cochrane collaboration, which had become a repository of information on safe and effective practice. Some of the problems with this direction for counsellors seemed related to the science itself (see Cooper and Reeves 2012), but also how EBP had been used against counsellors' normal and preferred ways of practice (Busch 2012). Specifically, the standardized diagnostic and treatment protocols developed in experimental conditions (e.g. CBT; Pearce 2014) often didn't align with counsellors' preferred approaches or fit client circumstances.

Some might wonder if counsellors shouldn't just chuck their "unproven" practices and approaches, and embrace those interventions legitimized by social science. EBP has been a highly contested professional expectation for some time in the US (Levant 2005) and in Canada (Dozois et al. 2014)—*among psychologists*. Part of the contest relates to the presumed transportability of "gold standard" research methods from medicine (see Goldacre 2010, 2013; Timmermans and Berg 2003) to evaluate the hard-to-standardize interventions of counselling, as previously discussed. However, another contested aspect of EBP relates to different stances on meaning and meaning-making, particularly by counsellors who self-identify as social constructionist (Paré 2013) or constructivist (Neimeyer and Raskin 2000). For these counsellors, different understandings of concerns and evidence are often turned to, to track client-preferred change, and to enable client feedback (i.e. practice-based evidence (PBE)) to inform the counselling process (Duncan, et al. 2004; Green and Latchford 2012). Counsellors have been less engaged in the evidence-based discussion than psychologists or psychiatric professionals, but the discussion is difficult for them avoid (see Yates 2013) when they are working in mental health services.

One development in the evidence-based discussion merits reflection: the growing use of neuroscience evidence to inform practice. While the DSM-5 has been found wanting by those preferring to ground research of mental health practice in neuroscience (see Insel 2013, but also Paris and Kirmayer 2016), the practice world has been abuzz for the past decade (circa 2007) regarding how neuroscience evidence justifies different clinical activities (see Boltanski and Thévenot 2006). Might neuroscience offer psychology a new uber-discourse, evidence by which one can understand what is really going on in terms of human concerns and changes associated with them, Stam (2015) mused recently? Neuroscience has provoked considerable debate regarding what it brings to the EBP discussion (Pitts-Taylor 2016). It is important to keep in mind that the brain pictures on which it is based do not directly address some important aspects in counselling like meaning and intention (Dumit 2004). Brains and brain parts alone are also not the source of human agency; they take up their respective contributions in human processes much like any other body part (Coulter 1979). Still, there has been something particularly compelling about neuroscience discourse for explaining human conduct (Ortega and Vidal 2011), prompting new forms of social science premised on neuropsychology informing an evidence base by which to manage the mind (Rose and Abi-Rached 2013).

In counselling, "neurobiology" knowledge and evidence has also become popular for providing a way of accounting for concerns and justifying the use of many interventions (e.g. Siegel 2012). It is unclear what an evidence-based based approach to the conversational work of counselling-based Research Domain criteria will mean, but neuroscience will likely justify conversational practices of diagnosing and treating mental disorders according to a very different science and evidence base (Hershenberg and Goldfried 2015; Insel 2013).

Legitimizing an Emerging Monoculture?

The title of this chapter, "Legitimizing an Emergent Mental Health "Monoculture"?," might seem an over-the-top choice of words I now need to justify. Throughout this chapter, I have been tracing counselling's development as a distinctive profession while it pursued ways to legitimize its members' services. Beginning as a vocation that took upon itself the task of guiding educational and career development, before moving on more broadly to help address human problems and difficulties, counselling was a field in which practitioners understandably sought greater professional legitimacy. It should not be surprising then, that the same year counsellors formed the American Personnel and Guidance Association (Leahy et al. 2015) was the year that the American Psychological Association established Division 17: Counseling Psychology to address human concerns considered less severe than those seen by clinical psychologists (Gladding 2013). A pecking order of sorts can be seen to emerge among non-psychiatrists in what would become mental health.

The funding of community mental health centers in the early 1960s required more mental health professionals to staff them, and that meant counsellors, as well as psychologists, social workers, and psychiatric nurses. Mental health took on broader connotations in the 1960s as new counselling approaches focused on the growth of human potential. Psychiatry itself had an image problem in the 1970s, and movement from the psychoanalytically focused nosology of DSM-II to the atheoretical symptom cluster focus of DSM-III was seen as a way of modernizing and legitimizing that profession (Frances 2013). Research into the effectiveness of prescription medications for treating DSM-III's diagnosed disorders accelerated for newly developing psychological interventions. The notion of an "emerging monoculture" derives from a concern about the centrality of medicalizing discourse for counselling given an enduring ambivalence regarding psychiatric diagnoses and EBP (e.g. Cooper and McLeod 2011).

"Emerging monoculture" may seem an overwrought phrase, conveying an odious sense of expected singularity where evidence to the contrary regarding counselling's "cultures of healing" (Cooper and McLeod 2011; Fancher 1995) persists. Even in a recent Delphi study, profession leaders cited a range of future aspirations for counselling, while positioning assistance on mental health issues as a top-ranked aim (Kaplan, et al. 2014). Legitimizing the profession and practice of counselling has entailed more than emulating developments in psychiatry and psychology. This is obvious when one traces the evolution of counsellors' professional identity (Gale and Austin 2003) and accreditation requirements for counsellor education programs (e.g. Robertson and Borgen 2016), as well as its licensing procedures (Lawson 2016). However, to work in mental health is to abide by its administrative expectations, and the mental health service, whether for publicly funded (Dozois et al. 2014) or privately managed (Reed and Eisman 2006) care, seldom advocates services offered in ways inconsistent with the current evidence-based public (EBP) rhetoric. Cost containment for such services tends to mean that counselling services are offered and managed as health-care services.

As Tanenbaum (2003: 295) has suggested, "Some of EBP's rhetorical potency comes from its ambiguity," and, at its most excessive, it stops being about informing practitioners and shifts to expected and stringent adherence to diagnostic and treatment protocols: a kind of professional script-following (Tanenbaum 2013). This would be a caricature of what some prefer to characterize as evidence-informed practice (Chwalisz 2003; Feltham 2005) while others have raised concerns about a potential EBP clinical overreach to administratively ensure treatment fidelity (Hagemoser 2009; Nelson et al. 2006). One version of a mental health "monoculture" that motivated this chapter relates to what some describe as a commodification of mental health disorders and evidence-based treatments (see Lakoff 2005, on pharmaceutical companies doing this, but also see Esposito and Perez 2014). The concern takes on a particular urgency as human services are increasingly privatized, while what I have been describing as medicalizing discourse comes to undergird rationing of services like counselling (cf. Abramovitz and Zelnick 2015). The evidence-based direction has provided counsellors with a basis to legitimize their ways of practice, bringing them in line with other mental health professionals, while such an alignment has perhaps caused some professional identity confusion at times (Gazzola and Smith 2007). To what extent must counselling's legitimacy be based on EBP?

Legitimizing counselling practice through this medicalizing direction has sometimes put the profession at odd with its traditions, partly over the role counsellors are to play in delivering services associated with "mental health," a term with broader medicalized connotations. For feminist scholars Lafrance and McKenzie-Mohr (2013), the DSM brings a "lure of legitimacy" to human concerns, and when conjoined with EBP conveys an algorithmic sense of professional practice that can be institutionally audited in training and research contexts as well as on the front lines of practice (Shore 2008). What brought things closer to what I have been terming a monoculture is the financial side of the work, and what it means to get paid by public and other third-party insurers. Outside of those systems of care where funding is not tied to the public purse or to private rationers, pluralism continues in counselling, and clients who can afford the service pay out of their own pocket. This is not the direction for counselling envisioned in the mid-twentieth century, but may become more likely in a post-Brexit, Trump-era economy.

References

Abbott, A. (1988). *The system of professions: An essay on the division of expert labor*. Chicago: University of Chicago Press.

Abramovitz, M., & Zelnick, J. (2015). Privatization in the human services: Implications for direct practice. *Clinical Social Work Journal, 43*(3), 283–293.

Alberti, R., & Emmons, M. (1970). *Your perfect right: A guide to assertive living*. Atascadero, CA: Impact.

Aubrey, R. F. (1977). Historical development of guidance and counseling and implications for the future. *Personnel and Guidance Journal, 55*(6), 288–295.

Aubrey, R. F. (1983). The odyssey of counseling and images of the future. *Personnel and Guidance Journal, 62*(2), 78–82.

Bandura, A. (1969). *Principles of behavior modification*. New York: Holt, Rinehart & Winston.

Berman, J. S., & Norton, N. C. (1985). Does professional training make a therapist more effective? *Psychological Bulletin, 98*(2), 401–407.

Boltanski, L., & Thévenot, L. (2006). *On justification: Economies of worth*. Princeton: Princeton University Press.

Bordin, E. S. (1979). The generalizability of the psychoanalytic concept of the working alliance. *Psychotherapy: Theory, Research & Practice, 16*(3), 252–260.

Borrelli, B., Sepinwall, D., Ernst, D., et al. (2005). A new tool to assess treatment fidelity and evaluation of treatment fidelity across 10 years of health behavior research. *Journal of Consulting and Clinical Psychology, 73*(5), 852–860.

Boston Women's Health Collective. (1971). *Our bodies, ourselves*. Boston: New England Free Press.

Busch, L. (2011). *Standards: Recipes for reality*. Cambridge, MA: MIT Press.

Busch, R. (2012). Problematizing social context in evidence-based therapy evaluation practice/governance. In A. Lock & T. Strong (Eds.), *Discursive perspectives in therapeutic practices* (pp. 245–268). Oxford: Oxford University Press.

Carkhuff, R. R. (1969). *Helping and human relations: A primer for professional leaders, Vol. 1: Selection and Training*. New York: Holt, Rinehart & Winston.

Carkhuff, R. R. (1972). *The art of helping*. Amherst, MA: Human Resource Development Press.

Cartwright, N., & Hardie, J. (2012). *Evidence-based policy: A practical guide to doing it better*. Oxford: Oxford University Press.

Chambless, D. L., & Hollon, S. D. (1998). Defining empirically supported therapies. *Journal of Consulting and Clinical Psychology, 66*(1), 7–18.

Chwalisz, K. (2003). Evidence-based practice: A framework for twenty-first century scientist-practitioner training. *The Counseling Psychologist, 31*(5), 497–528.

Cooper, M., & McLeod, J. (2011). *Pluralistic counselling and psychotherapy*. Thousand Oaks, CA: Sage.

Cooper, M., & Reeves, A. (2012). The role of randomised controlled trials in developing an evidence base for counselling and psychotherapy. *Counselling and Psychotherapy Research, 12*(4), 303–307.

Corey, G. (2016). *Theory and practice of counseling and psychotherapy* (10th ed.). Boston: Cengage Learning.

Coulter, J. (1979). The brain as agent. *Human Studies, 2*(1), 335–348.

Cumming, E. (1962). A review article: The reports of the joint commission on mental illness and health. *Social Problems, 9*(4), 391–400.

Cushman, P. (1995). *Constructing the self, constructing America: A cultural history of psychotherapy*. Boston: Da Capo Press.

Davis, J. (1914). *Vocational and moral guidance*. Boston: Ginn.

De Cicco, M. (n.d.). *Communication strategy plan with regard to the CCA name change*. Accessed from http://www.ccpa-accp.ca/_documents/CommunicationStrategy.pdf.
Downing, R. (2011). *Biohealth: Beyond medicalization: Imposing health*. Eugene, OR: Pickwick.
Dozois, D. J. A., Mikail, S. F., Alden, et al. (2014). The CPA presidential task force on evidence-based practice of psychological treatments. *Canadian Psychology, 55*(3), 153.
Dumit, J. (2004). *Picturing personhood: Brain scans and biomedical identity*. Princeton: Princeton University Press.
Duncan, B. L., Miller, S. D., & Sparks, J. A. (2004). *The heroic client: A revolutionary way to improve effectiveness through client-directed, outcome-informed therapy*. San Francisco: Jossey-Bass.
Ehrenwald, J. (Ed.). (1991). *The history of psychotherapy*. Northvale, NJ: Jason Aronson.
Eriksen, K., & Kress, V. E. (2006). The DSM and the professional counseling identity: Bridging the gap. *Journal of Mental Health Counseling, 28*(3), 202–217.
Esposito, L., & Perez, F. M. (2014). Neoliberalism and the commodification of mental health. *Humanity & Society, 38*(4), 414–442.
Fairclough, N. (1992). *Discourse and social change*. Cambridge: Polity Press.
Fancher, R. T. (1995). *Cultures of healing: Correcting the image of American mental health*. New York: W.H. Freeman.
Feltham, C. (2005). Evidence-based psychotherapy and counselling in the UK: Critique and alternatives. *Journal of Contemporary Psychotherapy, 35*(1), 131–143.
Ferguson, M. (1980). *The aquarian conspiracy: Personal and social transformation in our time*. Los Angeles: J.P. Tarcher.
Foucault, M. (1978). *Discipline and punish: The birth of the prison*. New York: Pantheon Books.
Foucault, M. (2003). *Psychiatric power: Lectures at the Collège de France, 1973–1974*. New York: Picador.
Frances, A. (2013). *Saving normal: An insider's revolt against out-of-control psychiatric diagnosis, DSM-5, big pharma, and the medicalization of ordinary life*. New York: William Morrow.
Frank, G. (1984). The Boulder Model: History, rationale, and critique. *Professional Psychology: Research and Practice, 15*(3), 417–435.

Furedi, F. (2004). *Therapy culture: Cultivating vulnerability in an uncertain age*. New York: Routledge.
Gale, A. U., & Austin, B. D. (2003). Professionalism's challenges to professional counselors' collective identity. *Journal of Counseling & Development, 81*(1), 3–10.
Gazzola, N., & Smith, D. J. (2007). Who do we think we are? A survey of counsellors in Canada. *International Journal for the Advancement of Counselling, 29*(2), 97–110.
Gladding, S. T. (2013). *Counseling: A comprehensive profession* (7th ed.). Upper Saddle River, NJ: Pearson.
Goffman, I. (1961). *Asylums: Essays on the social situation of mental patients and other inmates*. New York: Doubleday Anchor.
Goldacre, B. (2010). *Bad science: Quacks, hacks, and big pharma flacks*. New York: Farrar, Straus & Giroux.
Goldacre, B. (2013). *Bad pharma: How drug companies mislead doctors and harm patients*. New York: Farrar, Straus & Giroux.
Green, D., & Latchford, G. (2012). *Maximising the benefits of psychotherapy: A practice-based evidence approach*. West Sussex: Wiley-Blackwell.
Hacking, I. (1995). The looping effects of human kinds. In D. Sperber & A. J. Premack (Eds.), *Causal cognition* (pp. 351–383). Oxford: Oxford University Press.
Hage, S. M. (2003). Reaffirming the unique identity of counseling psychology: Opting for the 'Road less traveled by'. *The Counseling Psychologist, 31*(5), 555–563.
Hagemoser, S. D. (2009). Braking the bandwagon: Scrutinizing the science and politics of empirically supported therapies. *Journal of Psychology, 143*(6), 601–614.
Hartung, P. J., & Blustein, D. L. (2002). Reason, intuition, and social justice: Elaborating on Parsons's career decision-making model. *Journal of Counseling & Development, 80*(1), 41–47.
Havighurst, R. J. (1952). *Developmental tasks and education*. New York: Longmans, Green.
Hershenberg, R., & Goldfried, M. R. (2015). Implications of RDoC for the research and practice of psychotherapy. *Behavior Therapy, 46*(2), 156–165.
Hoffnung, R. J. (1969). Conditioning and transfer of affective self-references in a role-played counseling interview. *Journal of Consulting and Clinical Psychology, 33*(5), 527–531.
Holland, J. L., Magoon, T. M., & Magoon, A. R. (1981). Counseling psychology: Career interventions, research, and theory. *Annual Review of Psychology, 32*(1), 279–305.

House, R. (2004). *Therapy beyond modernity: Deconstructing and transcending profession-centred therapy*. London: Karnac.

Illouz, E. (2008). *Saving the modern soul: Therapy, emotions, and the culture of self-help*. Berkeley: University of California Press.

Insel, T. (2013). *Post by former NIMH director Thomas Insel: Transforming diagnosis*. Accessed November 18, 2016, from https://www.nimh.nih.gov/about/directors/thomas-insel/blog/2013/transforming-diagnosis.shtml.

Ivey, A. E., D'Andrea, M. J., & Ivey, M. B. (2011). *Theories of counseling and psychotherapy: A multicultural perspective* (7th ed.). London: Sage.

Jensen, P., Roper, M., Fisher, P., et al. (1995). Test-retest reliability of the Diagnostic Interview Schedule for Children (DISC 2.1): Parent, child, and combined algorithms. *Archives of General Psychiatry, 52*(1), 61–71.

Jevne, R. (1981). Counsellor competencies and selected issues in Canadian counsellor education. *Canadian Counsellor, 15*(2), 57–63.

Kaplan, D. M., Tarvydas, V. M., & Gladding, S. T. (2014). A vision for the future of counseling: The 20/20 principles for unifying and strengthening the profession. *Journal of Counseling and Development, 92*(3), 367–372.

Kesey, K. (1962). *One flew over the cuckoo's nest*. New York: Viking Press.

Kramer, U., & Stiles, W. B. (2015). The responsiveness problem in psychotherapy: A review of proposed solutions. *Clinical Psychology: Science and Practice, 22*(3), 277–295.

Kutchins, H., & Kirk, S. A. (2003). *Making us crazy: DSM: The psychiatric bible and the creation of mental disorders*. New York: Free Press.

Lafrance, M. N., & McKenzie-Mohr, S. (2013). The DSM and its lure of legitimacy. *Feminism & Psychology, 23*(1), 119–140.

Lakoff, A. (2005). *Pharmaceutical reason: Knowledge and value in global psychiatry*. Cambridge: Cambridge University Press.

Lawson, G. (2016). On being a profession: A historical perspective on counselor licensure and accreditation. *Journal of Counselor Leadership and Advocacy, 3*(2), 71–84.

Leahy, M. J., Rak, E., & Zanskas, S. A. (2015). A brief history of counseling and specialty areas of practice. In M. Stebnicki & I. Marini (Eds.), *Professional counselor's desk reference* (pp. 3–8). New York: Springer.

Levant, R. F. (2005). *Report of the 2005 presidential task force on evidence-based practice*. American Psychological Association. Accessed from https://www.apa.org/practice/resources/evidence/evidence-based-report.pdf.

Maslow, A. H. (1971). *The farther reaches of human nature*. New York: Viking Press.

Mathewson, R. H. (1949). *Guidance policy and practice*. New York: Harper.

Murray, H. A. (1938). *Explorations in personality*. New York: Oxford University Press.

Myers, D. (2007). Implication of the scientist-practitioner model in counseling psychology training and practice. *American Behavioral Scientist, 50*(6), 789–796.

Neimeyer, R. A., & Raskin, J. D. (Eds.). (2000). *Constructions of disorder: Meaning-making frameworks for psychotherapy*. Washington: American Psychological Association.

Nelson, T. D., Steele, R. G., & Mize, J. A. (2006). Practitioner attitudes toward evidence-based practice: Themes and challenges. *Administration and Policy in Mental Health and Mental Health Services Research, 33*(3), 398–409.

Nichols, M. P., & Schwartz, R. C. (2008). *Family therapy: Concepts and methods* (8th ed.). Boston: Pearson Allyn & Bacon.

Ogunfowora, B., & Drapeau, M. (2008). Comparing counselling and clinical psychology professionals: Similarities and differences on theoretical orientations revisited. *International Journal for the Advancement of Counselling, 30*(2), 93–103.

Online Etymology Dictionary. (n.d.). *Therapy*. Accessed November 21, 2016. http://www.etymonline.com/index.php?term=therapy.

Ortega, F., & Vidal, F. (Eds.). (2011). *Neurocultures: Glimpses into an expanding universe*. Frankfurt am Main: Peter Lang.

Paré, D. (2013). *The practice of collaborative counseling and psychotherapy: Developing skills in culturally mindful helping*. Los Angeles: Sage.

Paris, J., & Kirmayer, L. J. (2016). The National Institute of Mental Health research domain criteria: A bridge too far. *Journal of Nervous and Mental Disease, 204*(1), 26–32.

Pearce, P. (2014). Forty years on from Rogers' APA address 'Some new challenges for the helping professions. *Self & Society, 41*(2), 38.

Peavy, V., Robertson, S., & Westwood, M. (1982). Guidelines for counselor education in Canada. *Canadian Counselor, 16*(3), 135–143.

Perls, F. S. (1969). *Gestalt therapy verbatim*. Gouldsboro: The Gestalt Journal Press.

Pitts-Taylor, V. (2016). *The brain's body: Neuroscience and corporeal politics*. Durham, NC: Duke University Press.

Postle, D. (2007). *Regulating the psychological therapies: From taxonomy to taxidermy* (2nd ed.). Ross-on-Wye: PCCS Books.

Proctor, G. (2002). *The dynamics of power in counselling and psychotherapy: Ethics, politics and practice*. Ross-on-Wye: PCCS Books.

Proctor, W. M., Benefield, W., & Wrenn, C. G. (1931). *Workbook in vocations.* Boston: Houghton Mifflin.

Reed, G. M., & Eisman, E. J. (2006). Uses and misuses of evidence: Managed care, treatment guidelines, and outcome measurement in professional practice. In C. D. Goodheart, A. E. Kazdin, & R. J. Sternberg (Eds.), *Evidence-based psychotherapy: Where practice and research meet* (pp. 13–35). Washington: American Psychological Association.

Ringer, R. J. (1977). *Looking out for #1.* New York: Funk & Wagnalls.

Robertson, S. E., & Borgen, W. A. (2016). CCPA accreditation of counsellor education programs in Canada: An historical perspective/L'accréditation par l'ACCP des programmes de formation des conseillers au Canada: Une perspective historique. *Canadian Journal of Counselling and Psychotherapy (Online), 50*(3), 259.

Rogers, C. (1941). *Counseling and psychotherapy: Newer concepts in practice.* New York: Houghton Mifflin.

Rose, N. (1979). The psychological complex: Mental measurement and social administration. *Ideology and Consciousness, 5,* 5–68.

Rose, N., & Abi-Rached, J. M. (2013). *Neuro: The new brain sciences and the management of the mind.* Princeton: Princeton University Press.

Rosen, R. D. (1978). *Psychobabble: Fast talk and quick cure in the era of feeling.* New York: Atheneum.

Sampson, E. E. (1977). Psychology and the American ideal. *Journal of Personality and Social Psychology, 35*(11), 767–782.

Schutz, W. C. (1967). *Joy: Expanding human awareness.* New York: Grove Press.

Sennett, R. (1981). *Authority.* New York: Vintage.

Shapin, S. (2008). *The scientific life: A moral history of a late modern vacation.* Chicago: University of Chicago Press.

Shlien, J. M., & Zimring, F. M. (1966). Research directives and methods in client-centered therapy. In L. A. Gottshalk & A. H. Auerback (Eds.), *Methods of research in psychotherapy* (pp. 424–447). New York: Appleton Century Crofts.

Shore, C. (2008). Audit culture and illiberal governance: Universities and the politics of accountability. *Anthropological Theory, 8*(3), 278–298.

Siegel, D. J. (2012). *Pocket guide to interpersonal neurobiology: An integrative handbook of the mind.* New York: W.W. Norton.

Skinner, B. F. (1972). *Beyond freedom and dignity.* Harmondsworth: Penguin Books.

Spiegel, A. (2005, January 3). The dictionary of disorder. *The New Yorker*. Accessed November 17, 2016 http://www.newyorker.com/magazine/2005/01/03/the-dictionary-of-disorder.
Stam, H. J. (2015). The neurosciences and the search for a unified psychology: The science and esthetics of a single framework. *Frontiers in Psychology, 6,* 1467.
Steiner, C. (2012). *Automate this: How algorithms came to rule our world*. New York: Penguin.
Stiles, W. B., & Shapiro, D. A. (1989). Abuse of the drug metaphor in psychotherapy process-outcome research. *Clinical Psychology Review, 9*(4), 521–543.
Tanenbaum, S. (2003). Evidence-based practice in mental health: Practical weaknesses meet political strengths: Evidence-based practice in mental health. *Journal of Evaluation in Clinical Practice, 9*(2), 287–301.
Tanenbaum, S. J. (2013). Reducing variation in health care: The rhetorical politics of a policy idea. *Journal of Health Politics, Policy and Law, 38*(1), 5–26.
Timmermans, S., & Berg, M. (2003). *The gold standard: The challenge of evidence-based medicine and standardization in health care*. Philadelphia: Temple University Press.
Truax, C. B., & Carkhuff, R. (1967). *Toward effective counseling and psychotherapy: Training and practice*. Chicago: Aldine.
Tucker, A. R., & Blythe, B. (2008). Attention to treatment fidelity in social work outcomes: A review of the literature from the 1990s. *Social Work Research, 32*(3), 185–190.
VandenBos, G. R., Cummings, N. A., & DeLeon, P. H. (1992). A century of psychotherapy: Economic and environmental influences. In D. K. Freedheim (Ed.), *History of psychotherapy: A century of change* (pp. 65–102). Washington: American Psychological Association.
Whitaker, R. (2010). *Anatomy of an epidemic: Magic bullets, psychiatric drugs and the astonishing rise of mental illness*. New York: Broadway Paperbacks.
Wilson, M. (1993). DSM-III and the transformation of American psychiatry: A history. *American Journal of Psychiatry, 150*(3), 399–410.
Wolpe, J. (1958). *Psychotherapy by reciprocal inhibition*. Stanford: Stanford University Press.
Wrenn, G. (1962). *The counselor in a changing world*. Washington: American Personnel and Guidance Association.
Yates, C. (2013). Evidence-based practice: The components, history, and process. *Counseling Outcome Research and Evaluation, 4*(1), 41–54.
Young, R. A., & Lalande, V. (2011). Canadian counselling psychology: From defining moments to ways forward. *Canadian Psychology, 52,* 248–255.

5

Individualizing and Socializing the Mental Health Monoculture

With respect to psychologisation, one should not focus on the supposed real life behind it, but in reality show how life gets psychologised.
(De Vos 2012: 10)

Counselling, as I have been suggesting, has acquired some of its professional legitimacy by adopting the medicalizing discourse and research-associated practices of psychiatry and psychology. The confluence of medicine and psychology to address human concerns has been accelerating as new technologies and therapies enable people to overcome a range of upsets, irritations, and miseries others formerly put up with (see Davies 2015). In society at large, reference to a quality of life seems increasingly understood in terms borrowed from mental health, or by the more euphemistic term "wellness" (Cederström and Spicer 2015). Some sociologists and critical psychologists have been raising concerns that a therapy culture (Furedi 2004; Newnes 2011) has been on the rise and that a particular form of identity politics is emerging based on terms from what I have been describing as medicalizing discourse (McLaughlin 2012; Prince 2008). To read Cushman's (1995) historical account of the relationship between psychotherapy

T. Strong, *Medicalizing Counselling*, Palgrave Studies in the Theory and History of Psychology, DOI 10.1007/978-3-319-56699-3_5

and changing notions of selfhood is one way to relate to de Vos' quote at the beginning of this chapter. Another way is to ponder how concerns in the interpersonal or social realm get translated into diagnosable mental disorders needing treatment or self-management (House 2010; Rose 1997). In this Chap. 1 contend that the concerns clients bring to counselling owe something to how those concerns (and what can be done about them) have been mirrored back in the media by our mental health culture. To join counsellors in a mental health culture that legitimizes their practices, clients also had to act in ways consistent with mental health culture.

Following Foucault's studies into "mental health" (1968, 2008b), a critical psychology literature has developed and found a wide readership. Central to this literature is the notion that mental health, psychopathology, and mental health practices need to be understood as culturally and historically situated projects. Along similar lines for critical psychologists (see Parker 2015), attention needs to focus on the role that shifting cultural discourses play in articulating our concerns while shaping responses to them. Relatedly, "social pathologies" can be seen to provide contexts in which psychopathologies, or DSM-5 diagnosable disorders, find their expression (Keohane and Petersen 2013). New "identity cultures" based on such social pathologies can be seen to emerge (Brinkmann 2016), while new diagnoses are proposed and professionally taken up. The DSM-5 proposed criteria for "Internet Gaming Disorder" (APA 2013: 795) around the same time as gaming machine designers were finding new ways to target user vulnerabilities (Dow Schüll 2012). Thus, mental health and research respond to evolving concerns produced by some cultural developments, while turning inattentive to others that lose their cultural salience, echoing Shorter's (2013) musing about the disappearance of "nervous breakdowns."

For Ian Hacking (1995b, 1999), social pathologies find their diagnosable expression and related treatment through scientific knowledge taking root in particular cultural or "ecological niches" (1999). For example, he attributed what was formerly known as MPD to memory science, counselling approaches (particularly hypnoanalysis, and treatments associated with reclaiming memories of childhood sexual abuse), media uptake of MPD (movies like *Sybil* and the *Three Faces of Eve*), as well as “self-help” books and biographies. In other words, people could learn about themselves (e.g. that they may have been abused in satanic rituals) from such sources that, for Shorter (1992), offered disorder-related “templates” for making sense of otherwise ambiguous concerns, which then shaped how they could present their concerns meaningfully to others. Hacking (1999) later turned to a different ecological niche to study “fugue states” in late nineteenth-century Europe, in his *Mad Travelers*.

Situating and historicizing our social pathologies and mental disorders can help us make sense of the concerns clients bring to counsellors. My specific interest here is with trying to understand how developments associated with psychologizing and medicalizing discourses relate to concerns clients bring to counsellors. Hacking’s “looping effects” from medicalizing discourse are not only being mirrored back by clients, they are further reified through popularization in the public media (see Illouz 2008), constraints associated with health reimbursement procedures (Daniels 2001), and even through the quality of workplace initiatives (e.g. Csiernik and Csiernik 2012). Cultures also strategically and educationally target cultivating particular kinds of selves based on changing values and concerns (Martin and McLellan 2013); such concerns do not arise out of a cultural vacuum. For the philosopher Gilles Deleuze, such concerns stabilize in varied assemblages of meaning, interaction, and material reality (Deleuze and Guattari 1987; Duff 2014). Clients and counsellors can similarly become stuck in health-care assemblages (Duff 2014) through the understandings and responses they bring to contemporary cultural concerns.

There are varying views on how a mental health monoculture might look or take form. One dystopian version would update Aldous Huxley’s (1932) *Brave New World*, regarding optimal human existence as needing precision pharmaceutical management (see Lakoff 2005; Moncrieff 2008). Counselling increasingly means seeing clients on prescription medications, for whom the relative benefits of counselling and medications may be a mystery. Another technological component of managing one’s mental health is personalized mental health apps. Such apps have been evaluated for their potential usefulness as adjuncts to counselling on one hand (Hilty et al. 2016), and potentially insidious self-governance tools on the other (Rich and Miah 2017). Developments in psychopharmacology and personal mental health technologies will be the focus of the chapter, but these are not the only contributors to extending and further reifying potentials for a mental health monoculture.

Consistent with these and other evolving facets of mental health culture is an increased focus on symptom monitoring and relief, alongside a more aspirational focus on optimizing one's potentials as valued capabilities and "wellness" (Cederström and Spicer 2015). The boundaries between relieving one's symptoms and enhancing one's wellness may seem to be flipsides of the same coin. However, the WHO's definition of health since 1948 has been: "Health is a state of complete physical, mental and social well-being and not merely the absence of disease or infirmity" (WHO 2003). How health gets defined and correspondingly addressed matters to critics, such as Duff (2014), for whom current definitions have excessively focused on a personalized, skin-encapsulated, subjective view. Part of my focus in this chapter is to examine the limitations of this individualized view.

Health and especially mental health has become a focus of critical concern, particularly since Foucault's critical writing (1968, 1973), and early sociological studies that examined social processes and language use associated with health (e.g. Scheff 1967). There is a longstanding critique pertaining to the role that mental health knowledge and its applications can play in subjectivizing injustices that might otherwise be understood as social, institutional, or societal (e.g. Brown 2006; Ingleby 1980; Smith and Siegel 1985). The gist of the critique is that counsellors and mental health professionals using such knowledge turn attention inward and downplay or avoid the significance of what is externally affecting clients' lives. This focus inward takes many forms, but is consistent with psychology's general focus on brains and skin-encapsulated individuals. Since counselling has heavily drawn on psychology as its primary discourse of understanding and evidence, the social, institutional, and cultural aspects of clients' lives have traditionally received less consideration, though this has been changing (e.g. Audet and Paré 2017; Monk et al. 2008). This individualizing focus in mental health is consistent with Conrad's (2007) medicalizing logic of diagnosis and treatment, with one added dimension: a self-*management* imperative (Rose 1990, 1997) is added to the logic. The critical question scholars raise is: on whose terms is this self-management done (e.g. Rose 1990)?

Managing one's mental health could be equated with other forms of self-management, be that managing a professional identity, a budget, or one's time (see Burkeman 2016). The metaphor of management suggests deploying forms of knowledge and guidelines (Pinder and Bourgeois 1982) to optimize particular benefits and minimize unwanted outcomes—in this case, pertaining to one's mental health. These optimized "mental health benefits" relate to what Taylor (1997: 145) has referred to as social goods that somehow merge with individual virtues: "As long as you think that all goods must be individual, and that any other construal is incoherent, you can't see there is a moral argument here." This was Danziger's (1997) observation; that our psychological vocabularies were often imported from moral discourse. Thus, "managing" one's expected conduct and mental health tends to be done on bases that can vary as "social goods" or morals, a basis found in and applicable to counselling's history as well (Cushman 1995).

It is the convergence of personal and public understandings of such management efforts pertaining to mental health that are of interest here. Psychology supplies morally laden constructs such as self-actualization, "executive functioning," values, identity, and esteem (see de Vos 2012) that seem amenable to a management focus, whether through forms of self-discipline (Foucault 2010; Miller and Rose 2008) or as facilitated by mental health professionals (e.g. Sampson 1981; Sflakidou and Kefalopoulou 2015). As the expert language of DSM-5 and EBP found its way into the popular vocabularies and understandings of the public, mental health discourse has been increasingly implicated in the understandings and self-management projects of the public (Furedi 2004; Illouz 2008). By Furedi's account, ours is a therapy culture, one which is becoming increasingly vulnerable and enfeebled (Gergen 1990). By such a medicalizing logic and its cultural uptake, people require greater amounts of mental health assistance and attend more to their vulnerabilities and psychiatric symptoms than to the kinds of resilience that purportedly got earlier generations through trying times (Furedi 2004). Many counsellors who favor strengths-based and resiliency-focused approaches (e.g. Duncan et al. 2004) would struggle with Furedi's sociological account, but these counsellors would not represent those with mainstream mental health understandings circulating in the public domain.

Eva Illouz is another sociologist who has looked closely at relationships between the public media and "personal" understandings of the mental health kind, illustrating how "looping effects" (Hacking 1995a) culturally operate in effect. One of her early books was entitled *Oprah Winfrey and the Glamour of Misery: An Essay on Popular Culture* (Illouz 2003). For Illouz, our often inchoate emotional lives find new forms of recognition and expression through popularized portrayals of how feelings are to be understood, presented, and talked about. The confessional nature of celebrity interviews, for example, offer distillations of mental health understandings by those who have lived such mental health experiences as eating disorders, depression, and PTSD. This is a sociocultural view of how personal and public emotional lives come to be intertwined, how misery finds a linguistic handle and culturally appropriate and familiar means of expression. As Illouz later wrote directly in ways related to counselling and mental health, "We cannot separate the narratives of suffering from that of self-help and the thread connecting them are many and contradictory" (Illouz 2007: 62). Extending this observation to how clients may expectantly present, counsellors may feel compelled to join clients in mental health self-narratives and projects at odds with their preferred approaches to practice (Strong et al. 2015).

What Illouz and Furedi are pointing to is an emergence of recent culturally endorsed ways of understanding and showing one's experiences and understandings of suffering. What seemingly can resolve the "contradictoriness" Illouz raises is the kind of scientifically legitimized medical expertise found in the DSM-5 and related EBPs for treating its disorders. One might wonder how such expertise acquires a cultural cachet independent of its use by mental health professionals. The answer is that a self-help literature, based on professional help to others, has guided people's culturally and personally appropriate conduct for centuries (Starker 2002).

There can be a profession-serving (see House 2004) dismissal of such non-expert concerns as "folk psychology" (Ravenscroft 2016);

where scientific knowledge and public knowledge are seen to converge illegitimately, if not dangerously. A considerable debate has gone on among mental health professionals about what to do about clients' professed understandings of their concerns and what needs to be done about them. While some would see prospective clients as resourceful in their efforts to overcome concerns brought to counselling (Bohart and Tallman 1996; Duncan et al. 2004), the more conventional view is that the counsellor remains the expert in diagnosing and treating client concerns (Seligman 2004). Still, it should be no surprise that prospective clients make cyber-visits to Dr. Google (Murgia 2016) or PsychCentral (e.g. Grohol 2016) prior to coming for counselling. Such sites showcase how one's concerns can be symptomatically translated into medical discourse, finding further reinforcement at numerous blogs that personalized knowledge about "their diagnosis," including how to treat it and live with it (e.g. Krans 2016). The upshot is that there are innumerable resources people access to understand and share their concerns in a medicalized mental health discourse.

The parallels between medicalizing mental health discourse and psychological discourse as personal sources of expert knowledge should be apparent. There are commonalities between psychological knowledge and practice, and medical knowledge and practice, an intended aim in clinical psychology's move toward EBP (Chambless and Hollon 1998). Psychological knowledge tends to be normative, and so it is typically the unwanted abnormalities that compel the interests of those wanting to make use of such knowledge to better themselves or others. Bettering oneself involves addressing or measuring up to a "social good," in Taylor's (1997) sense. Psychology has generated many such goods, and notions of personhood have changed with them (Rose 1997). Nikolas Rose (1990, 1997) has examined such changing notions of personhood, less as personal pursuits of such "goods," and more as responses to cultural expectations, such as the need to develop "good" soldiers or industrial employees. More alarmingly, Rose is interested in how the state and its varied institutions specify and regulate subjectivity, the kinds of people we are "supposed to be." Psychology has played an important role in such specifying and regulating, mapping out developmental norms and the "tasks" required to meet them, providing management principles that optimize worker productivity, and grooming aspirants for future administrative roles. Tied to this assumed role for psychology has been the promise that its knowledge and practices would be appropriate for engineering particular kinds of people who learn to discipline or "govern" (Gergen 1990; Rose 1990) themselves in culturally and institutionally expected ways. Abnormalities can be disciplined back into normalities, while education systems can produce culturally expected "selves" (Martin and McLellan 2013).

People are, of course, not automatons in Rose's bleak view; but there is a demonstrable kind of coercion at work in the kinds of selves to be produced. An extreme version relates to Canada's abhorrent, historical use of education to acculturate First Nations Children—to stamp out the 2015 Indian in them (TRC). This is a stark example of how political problems were addressed through educational and psychological means; a recurring theme in the governmentality literature that followed Foucault's and later, Rose's writing (e.g. Hook 2007). Psychology has, for example, played a central role in addressing such thorny human issues as criminality, employability, parental ability, even dating profiles (Davies 2015; de Vos 2012). It is the scientific authority of psychology that has been the source of the disciplinary power to enable decisions, target wanted and unwanted social behaviors, and cultivate particular kinds of selves (Prilleltensky 1994).

Where psychology's role takes on an added heft, however, is through what it enables aspirationally, through the kinds of self-governing knowledge (governmentalities) Foucault and others have referred to as "biopower" (Hook 2007; Rose 1997). For biopower to be operative it must convey both a sense of the applied knowledge expected to address one's needs, but also should enable one to feel empowered to become the kind of person one ostensibly wants to be. My choice of the word ostensibly relates to how people align the person they want to be with the culturally desired psychological person they aim to cultivate and discipline. Governmentality refers to these culturally recognizable ways of managing oneself according to temporally shifting cultural ideals (i.e. goods) or norms (Dean 2013). Here is Foucault (2008a: 17), in one of his lectures, and playfully paraphrasing a famous line from Nietzsche, on the variability of that kind of person, that kind of "self-discipline":

"The state is nothing else but the mobile effect of a regime of multiple governmentalities." The psychological person we aim (or are) to become and self-discipline changes with these "governmentalities."

Bio-(Mental) Health Narratives and Technologies of the Self

> [T]echnologies of self… permit individuals to effect by their own means or with the help of others a certain number of operations on their own bodies and souls, thoughts, conduct, and any way of being, so-as-to-transform themselves in order to attain a certain state of happiness, purity, wisdom, perfection or immortality. (Foucault 1988: 18)

Psychology and the medicalizing discourse of mental health in effect provided not only professionals with a language for counselling, they made accessible to a curious public "grids of intelligibility" (Foucault 1990: 93) by which people could orient themselves, to find sense-making resources to understand their concerns and what can be done about them. Biopower is a central concept in the later lectures and writing of Michel Foucault (e.g. 2008a, b) and refers to people's self-applications of such biomedical knowledge to transform themselves in the manner Foucault suggests in the quote at the beginning of this section. Technologies of the self are the learnable and reproducible ways ("operations" for Foucault) by which people can "govern" or fashion lives based on knowledge such as that which comes from the medicalizing discourse of mental health.

Technologies of the self extend a view that human beings are "self-interpreting animals" (Taylor 1985). It is in this sense that we can understand people taking up "illness narratives" (see Frank 1995; Thompson 2012) to apply coherent and culturally familiar ways of making sense of their lives and to guide how they should act. In the colorful, self-published, language of Janet Byron Anderson (2012; Kindle Location 91), such medical conditions and stories take up "dual citizenship," passing for expert knowledge in both medical and popular media contexts. Illouz's (2003) celebrity confessionals offer such narratives, as do mental health blogs, and other accessible media which proliferate in mental health discourse—ready for self-application. Such narrative resources are hardly benign, the storylines arising from them "help" by informing how one should experience and address mental health concerns. They also showcase performable "technologies of the self" by which people can govern their concerns or discipline thoughts and actions accordingly. Being self-interpreting animals, humans often try to understand and act in culturally expected ways (Elias 1994) and this extends to their taking up cultural behaviors expected to empower them biomedically or psychologically (Hook 2007). By using mental health discourse, people become agents on their own behalf, or "good clients" (Gillett 2009).

Foucault's (2010) later lectures also foretold how mental health culture would come to feature in recent "governmentality" literature (e.g. Dean 2013; Hook 2007; Walters 2012). Part of Foucault's interest was with politics we now know as neoliberalism (Harvey 2005), and governmentality refers to how people manage the purported freedoms associated with neoliberalism. There can seem a counterintuitive point Foucault is raising, that people would *"govern" their freedom* in potentially slavish ways. Those steeped in the ideas of humanist psychology would struggle with this point. Humanist psychology was partly premised on the notion that there was a core authentic self (think of the metaphor of peeling away layers of the onion to get to ourselves as we essentially are) that could be the source of genuine desires and actions. Such a genuine or authentic self—when healthy—ostensibly could make personally congruent choices and was a self that was immortalized in Fritz Perls' (1969: 4) Gestalt prayer:

I do my thing and you do your thing.

I am not in this world to live up to your expectations,

And you are not in this world to live up to mine.

You are you, and I am I,

and if by chance we find each other, it's beautiful.

If not, it can't be helped.

Here is another 1960s icon, Carl Rogers, getting at a related humanist concept: "when the individual is inwardly free, he chooses as the good life, this process of becoming" (1961: 196). The self so central to humanist psychology was the self that Foucault (2005) critically took on, contending that our notions of selfhood did not emanate from *within* ourselves, but were related to our historical and cultural situatedness. Regardless, psychology's vocabulary of selfhood tends to be premised on a humanist and individualist view of our innate potential (Danziger 1997).

I have been describing a "romantic," humanist self, one ready for the modern knowledge psychology and mental health could provide for managing our freedom (Gergen 1991). This is the knowledge that our earlier discussed "grids of intelligibility" supply, to address an imperative Foucault (2005) identified for "care of the self." Such self-care, however, follows from how one cares for or "governs" others (Foucault 2005). To care for oneself or others means acquiring knowledge and practices suited for the task of caring for others *and* oneself, a broad challenge that has preoccupied psychology as a social science (Rose 1997). However, for Foucault (2005), psychology's knowledge and tasks cannot be universal as seemingly promised because it is not a natural science with knowledge applicable for *engineering* human outcomes (Richards 2010).

Foucault saw human concerns and aspirations as somewhat arbitrary or culturally relative, since situated living requires changing hermeneutics of self-making (see also Taylor 1989). Put differently, we understand and live our lives on different terms in different circumstances and there is no getting down to bottom of what is within our psyches: our subjectivity is interpretively derived from the cultural knowledge and values accessible within our circumstances. The notion of a genuine or true self, however, is often psychologized (de Vos 2012) and can inform an engineering logic associated with "technologies of the self" (Hook 2007). Instead of an "authentic" self hermeneutically grounded in historical and cultural context (Guignon 2004), a modern self, made knowable and changeable psychologically, can be targeted for transformation. In the 1990s, author Peter Kramer (1997) suggested that medications could enable designer personalities. Extending such a logic, technologies of the self, derived from psychological knowledge, should address human concerns as psychological concerns (Foucault 2008b;

Rose 1997). Mental health knowledge—psychological and medical—enables an intelligibility for governing oneself—apps, medications, and self-discipline extend this logic.

A question might arise as to how human concerns get translated onto coordinates associated with a mental health grid of intelligibility. Given that different discourses articulating such concerns (e.g. religious, social justice) are prevalent, why should human concerns most plausibly be understood in mental health terms? How does human attention and self-discipline get directed inward for concerns that might otherwise be directed outwardly? With good reason, many would respond that this doesn't always happen, and that one is free to base their well-being on other discourses in circulation, as if there was a marketplace of discourses. Mental health discourse tends to be more individual in focus, promoting subjective and somewhat neoliberal responses that some critics cite as "entrepreneurial" (Lazzarato 2014). Behind any responses to human concerns, however, is what justifies any response as appropriate or legitimate: understandings and responses we could justify to each other (Boltanski and Thévenot 2006).

Medicalization has enabled society to push back boundaries on what has been considered personally or socially acceptable (Conrad 2007; Clarke et al. 2010). For Illich, medicalization enabled greater personal autonomy, such that "health" can sometimes be considered "identical with lived freedom" (1977: 244). Whether diminishing disquiets or actualizing cherished potentials, medicalization has become a means to pursue both personal and cultural ends. The postmodern sociologist Zygmunt Bauman (2000) wrote of "identity projects," ways in which people fashion themselves in response to both adversity and what they desire in life. For Foucault (2008b), such "self-care" entails a three-step process, requiring: (a) observing (or learning about) how others get taken care of, (b) making oneself the object of such knowledge and care, and (c) subjecting (or disciplining) oneself according to what one has learned. Such "self-care," in other words, is justified on the basis of knowledge and practices deemed authoritative or legitimate (Sennett 1981) for producing particular subjectivities, like Bauman's identity projects. This is an approach to subjectivity and self-care tailor-made for a free market neoliberal culture (Cushman 1990; Harvey 2005).

Psychology's individualism and the presumption that individuals are consumers and entrepreneurs in a global free market converge in what might seem an unlikely confluence. For concerned scholars, like Miller and Rose (2008), this has been no coincidence: mental health knowledge and related scientific practices have become essential for governing oneself and others. In other words, it isn't only that the marketplace uses psychological knowledge to inform product development and marketing, the research methods of psychologists are now embedded in our technologies. For example, psychological research methods for identifying normative understandings and decisions now inform Web 2.0 algorithms that enable online merchants such as Amazon or iTunes to suggest purchases consistent with our purchasing patterns (Davies 2015; Steiner 2012). Relatedly, marketers have become more skilled in identifying and amplifying our concerns, while at the same time proposing tailored solutions to address those concerns (Morozov 2013; Toscano and Kinkle 2015). This is best exemplified by the ways in which medications to manage particular disorders (Conrad 2007) and relieve mental health symptoms are now advertised (Busfield 2010; Whitaker 2010).

Mental health knowledge is also now central to workplace and community efforts to optimize wellness (Cederström and Spicer 2015), and "smart devices" that promise happiness (Davies 2015). One can become a savvy consumer and assertive user of mental health apps (Dellabella n.d.) and a similarly assertive advocate regarding one's medication and counselling needs (Parikh 2015). Such self-advocacy in addressing one's mental health needs and aspirations requires knowledge appropriated from mental health science and practice. The disciplining aspects (i.e. technologies of the self) of a mental health kind of governmentality involve more than fickle consumerism or transient "solutionism" (Morozov 2013); particular kinds of surveillance and vigilance pertaining to self-care practices are required.

While today's mental health owes some of its origins to the mental hygiene movement (Cushman 1995), prevention-oriented as well as treatment-related self-care initiatives to promote a mental health governmentality are increasingly evident. There has been a growing "mental health literacy" movement, designed to help people self-monitor for a range of mental health symptoms and disorders (Jorm 2000). Depression screening, for example, is now commonplace and has been equated with routine medical check-ups (Ebeling 2011; Morey et al. 2015). A doctoral student working with me, Karen Ross, has been examining mental health concerns and wellness campaigns on post-secondary campuses (e.g. Lunau 2012; Rosenbaum and Liebert 2015; Stewart et al. 2014). On my campus this has been a fraught topic, as a year-end student party a few years ago ended with five fatal stabbings. Subsequently, a major new mental health initiative for students was launched (University of Calgary 2015). Especially interesting from Karen's research are the different discourses and media students turn to when making sense of and addressing their concerns (Nesi and Prinstein 2015; Steers et al. 2014). There is now "mental health first aid" on campuses, despite questions raised about the way such first aid might divert attention away from social justice issues (DeFehr 2016). More often than not, however, social justice in this respect has focused on stigma mitigation and legitimizing having a diagnosed mental disorder (e.g. Eisenberg et al. 2009). One particular variation on this social justice theme arose from people who had been formerly diagnosed in the DSM-IV with Asperger's syndrome, and losing what for them had been a distinctive, if not quirky, self-identification they embraced proudly (Giles 2014). Trauma identities and vulnerability ("triggers") are justified through citing relevant DSM-5 (McLaughlin 2012) diagnoses. To discuss many human concerns nowadays seems to require beginning from default discourses like those of mental health or wellness (Cederström and Spicer 2015).

Different kinds of "diagnostic cultures" (Brinkmann 2016) informing and normalizing what it means to "appropriately" live with a diagnosis of a mental disorder are a related cultural phenomenon. This points to another facet of medicalization, that goes beyond the kind of "diagnose and treat logic" (Conrad 2007) that has been our primary focus up until now. Specifically, many medicalized conditions are considered chronic, and so there is no treatment or cure. Instead there is symptom management (Clarke et al. 2010) and this also can require or invite identity changes such as assuming "disability status" and surrendering some degree of personal autonomy to the state, and one's health-care workers

(Moss and Teghtsoonian 2008). This, however, is also where new forms of governmentality can be summoned or expected, as those who have been diagnosed require new forms of self-vigilance or "self-care" (see Binkley 2011). It is not uncommon for people taking on diagnosis-based identities (e.g. McLaughlin 2012) to find themselves having to accommodate to new routines and self-care practices—in the kinds of "subjection" that Judith Butler (1997: 84) suggested comes with being both "acted upon" and "activated by" what comes with a diagnosis.

Counselling in a Self-Help World?

> The politics of recognition in interaction with wider political and social change, has become heavily focused on the fragility of the self, inherent vulnerability and susceptibility to psychological and physical harm. (McLaughlin 2012: 129)

From the outset, I have indicated that my interests in this book rest with human concerns that historically have not been medicalized: the most common being "sub-clinical" kinds of depression (Horwitz and Wakefield 2007) and anxiety (Horwitz and Wakefield 2012). But there are many other concerns that would not normally be seen as disorders, such as relational difficulties, non-complicated bereavement, vocational concerns, and so on. When I worked in a mental health center in the early 1990s these were the kinds of coping concerns that might be categorized as "adjustment disorders," so that clients could still be seen. These days, when people struggle to cope, it may not be surprising that their struggles are understood as being related to a mental disorder. There are ample opportunities for people to self-diagnose (Strong et al. 2015), relating their upsets and disquiets to symptom clusters associated with DSM-5 diagnoses, and to narratives offered by celebrity testimonials and personal blogs pertaining to diagnosed conditions. In the last generation, increasingly accessible mental health knowledge has informed people on how to monitor their bodies and minds, and engage in familiar forms of self-care to avoid *or* embrace mental health clienthood (Hook 2007).

Mental health "monoculture" is an admittedly excessive term for what I have been describing, particularly for that fuzzy zone of unwanted experience that might be translatable to a diagnosable mental disorder. Problems and difficulties, however, often won't get someone a funded visit with a counsellor these days (Moses 2000; Wylie 1995). As skyrocketing rates of psychiatric medication use suggest (Frances 2013; Whitaker 2010), people's concerns tend to be less conversed to resolution, and more drugged into symptom relief. A therapist, former client, and journalist who has carefully examined the fuzzy zone, Gary Greenberg (2010, 2013), has been tracing the DSM process up to the publication of the DSM-5. Depression in particular has been part of Greenberg's focus, and he described participating in drug trials, he also participated in the EBP, cognitive therapy. Thought modification in this approach was, for Greenberg, ideological in its can-do optimism (2010), and critiques of such positive thinking in the face of adversity have been around since it was touted as a strategy for growing rich (Hill 1937) or since Peale's (1952) evangelically toned volume: *The Power of Positive Thinking*. Promoting inner optimism as depression treatment is understandable though it plays into agendas critics see as diminishing the hardships and miseries endured in everyday life (e.g. Ehrenreich 2009). Recently, it also served as the basis for Lord Layard's (2005) cultural prescription that more happiness could address the nation's economic woes. Layard's prescription also translated into the eventual Improving Access to Psychological Therapies initiative that recommended cognitive therapy, given its status as an evidence-based therapy.

Throughout this Chap. 1 have been suggesting that a potential mental health monoculture has been both individualizing and socializing medicalizing discourse. I used the term "monoculture" because, for many, a diagnose, treat, and manage logic has become common sense, and central to how human concerns are appropriately understood and addressed. Given changes associated with the DSM-III to DSM-5 diagnostic classification systems, and evidence-based therapies based on these diagnoses, a mental health governmentality has emerged that promotes scientific approaches to both self-care and mental health service responses (Foucault 2008b; Hook 2007). Taking care of oneself and others on such a medicalizing basis has arguably become part of a culturally accepted norm in everyday conversations, self-understandings, and professional conversations (Miller and Rose 2008). While such developments have not totalized public discourse on human concerns (e.g. social justice, spiritual discourses still are cited; e.g. Chung and Bemak 2013), medicalizing discourse has been sedimenting into people's everyday understandings and responses to human concerns. While such discursive sedimentation tends to constrain the possibilities for alternatively understanding and responding to such concerns, this sedimentation will focus the reading in Chap. 6.

References

Anderson, J. B. (2012). *Sick English: Medicalization in the English Language* (Kindle DX version). Accessed from https://www.amazon.ca/Sick-English-Medicalization-Language-ebook/dp/B00AEH3BEQ.

APA (American Psychiatric Association). (2013). *Diagnostic and statistical manual of mental disorders* (5th ed.). Washington: Author.

Audet, C., & Paré, D. A. (Eds.). (2017). *Social justice and counselling*. New York: Routledge.

Bauman, Z. (2000). *Liquid modernity*. Malden: Blackwell.

Binkley, S. (2011). Psychological life as enterprise: Social practice and the government of neo-liberal interiority. *History of the Human Sciences, 24*(3), 83–102.

Bohart, A. C., & Tallman, K. (1996). The active client: Therapy as self-help. *Journal of Humanistic Psychology, 36*(3), 7–30.

Boltanski, L., & Thévenot, L. (2006). *On justification: Economies of worth*. Princeton: Princeton University Press.

Brinkmann, S. (2016). *Diagnostic cultures: A cultural approach to the pathologization of modern life*. London: Routledge.

Brown, L. S. (2006). Still subversive after all these years: The relevance of feminist therapy in the age of evidence-based practice. *Psychology of Women Quarterly, 30*(1), 15–24.

Burkeman, O. (2016, December 22). Why time management is ruining our lives. *The Guardian*. Accessed December 25, 2016, from https://www.theguardian.com/technology/2016/dec/22/why-time-management-is-ruining-our-lives?CMP=share_btn_fb.

Busfield, J. (2010). 'A pill for every ill': Explaining the expansion in medicine use. *Social Science and Medicine, 70*(6), 934–941.

Butler, J. (1997). *The psychic life of power: Theories in subjection*. Stanford: Stanford University Press.

Cederström, C., & Spicer, A. (2015). *The wellness syndrome*. Cambridge: Polity Press.

Chambless, D. L., & Hollon, S. D. (1998). Defining empirically supported therapies. *Journal of Consulting and Clinical Psychology, 66*(1), 7–18.

Clarke, A. E., Mamo, L., Fosket, J. R., Fishman, J. R., & Shim, J. K. (Eds.). (2010). *Biomedicalization: Technoscience, health and illness in the US*. Durham, NC: Duke University Press.

Conrad, P. (2007). *The medicalization of society*. Baltimore: Johns Hopkins University Press.

Csiernik, R., & Csiernik, A. (2012). Canadian employee assistance programming: An overview. *Journal of Workplace Behavioral Health, 27*(2), 100–116.

Cushman, P. (1990). Why the self is empty: Toward a historically situated psychology. *American Psychologist, 45*(5), 599–611.

Cushman, P. (1995). *Constructing the self, constructing America: A cultural history of psychotherapy*. Boston: Da Capo Press.

Daniels, J. A. (2001). Managed care, ethics, and counseling. *Journal of Counseling & Development, 79*(1), 119–122.

Danziger, K. (1997). *Naming the mind: How psychology found its language*. Thousand Oaks, CA: Sage.

Davies, W. (2015). *The happiness industry: How the government and big business sold Us well-being*. London: Verso.

De Vos, J. (2012). *Psychologisation in times of globalisation*. London: Routledge.

Dean, M. (2013). *The signature of power: Sovereignty, governmentality and biopolitics*. London: Sage.

DeFehr, J. N. (2016). Inventing mental health first aid: The problem of psychocentrism. *Studies in Social Justice, 10*(1), 18–35.

Deleuze, G., & Guattari, F. (1987). *A thousand plateaus: Capitalism and schizophrenia*. London: Continuum.

Dow Schüll, N. (2012). *Addiction by design: Machine gambling in Las Vegas*. Princeton: Princeton University Press.

Duff, C. (2014). *Assemblages of health: Deleuze's empiricism and the ethology of life*. London: Springer.

Duncan, B. L., Miller, S. D., & Sparks, J. A. (2004). *The heroic client: A revolutionary way to improve effectiveness through client-directed, outcome-informed therapy*. San Francisco: Jossey-Bass.

Ebeling, M. (2011). 'Get with the program!' Pharmaceutical marketing, symptom checklists and self-diagnosis. *Social Science and Medicine, 73*(6), 825–832.

Ehrenreich, B. (2009). *Bright-sided: How the relentless promotion of positive thinking has undermined America*. New York: Metropolitan Books.

Eisenberg, D., Downs, M. F., Golberstein, E., & Zivin, K. (2009). Stigma and help seeking for mental health among college students. *Medical Care Research and Review, 66*(5), 522–541.

Elias, N. (1994). *The civilizing process*. Oxford: Blackwell.

Foucault, M. (1968). *Madness and civilization: A history of insanity in the age of reason* (R. Howard, Trans). New York: Vintage.

Foucault, M. (1973). *The birth of the clinic: An archaeology of medical perception*. London: Tavistock.

Foucault, M. (1988). Technologies of the self. In L. H. Marin, H. Gutman, & P. H. Hutton (Eds.), *Technologies of the self: A seminar with Michel Foucault* (pp. 16–49). Amherst, MA: University of Massachusetts Press.

Foucault, M. (1990). An introduction. *The history of sexuality* (Vol. 1). New York: Random House.

Foucault, M. (2005). *The hermeneutics of the subject: Lectures at the Collège de France, 1981–1982*. New York: Picador.

Foucault, M. (2008a). *The birth of biopolitics: Lectures at the Collège de France, 1978–1979*. New York: Palgrave Macmillan.

Foucault, M. (2008b). *History of madness*. New York: Routledge.

Foucault, M. (2010). *The government of self and others: Lectures at the Collège de France, 1982–1983*. New York: Picador.

Frances, A. (2013). *Saving normal: An insider's revolt against out-of-control psychiatric diagnosis, DSM-5, big pharma, and the medicalization of ordinary life*. New York: William Morrow.

Frank, A. W. (1995). *The wounded storyteller: Body, illness, and ethics*. Chicago: University of Chicago Press.

Furedi, F. (2004). *Therapy culture: Cultivating vulnerability in an uncertain age*. New York: Routledge.

Gergen, K. J. (1990). Therapeutic professions and the diffusion of deficit. *Journal of Mind and Behavior, 11*(3–4), 353–368.

Gergen, K. J. (1991). *The saturated self: Dilemmas of identity in contemporary life*. New York: Basic Books.

Giles, D. C. (2014). 'DSM-V is taking away our identity': The reaction of the online community to the proposed changes in the diagnosis of Asperger's disorder. *Health, 18*(2), 179.

Gillett, G. (2009). *The mind and its discontents*. Oxford: Oxford University Press.

Greenberg, G. (2010). *Manufacturing depression: The secret history of a modern disease*. Toronto: Simon & Schuster.

Greenberg, G. (2013). *The book of woe: The DSM and the unmaking of psychiatry*. New York: Penguin.

Grohol, J. (2016). Symptoms and treatments of mental disorders. *Psych Central*. Accessed November 28, 2016, from http://psychcentral.com/disorders/.

Guignon, C. (2004). *On being authentic*. New York: Routledge.

Hacking, I. (1995a). *Rewriting the soul: Multiple personality and the sciences of memory*. Princeton: Princeton University Press.

Hacking, I. (1995b). The looping effects of human kinds. In D. Sperber & A. J. Premack (Eds.), *Causal cognition* (pp. 351–383). Oxford: Oxford University Press.

Hacking, I. (1999). *The social construction of what?* Cambridge, MA: Harvard University Press.

Harvey, D. (2005). *A brief history of neoliberalism*. Oxford: Oxford University Press.

Hill, N. (1937). *Think and grow rich*. Cleveland, OH: The Ralston Publishing Company.

Hilty, D. M., Yellowlees, P. M., Myers, K., Parish, M. B., & Rabinowitz, T. (2016). The effectiveness of e-mental health: Evidence base, how to choose the model based on ease/cost/strength, and future areas of research. In *E-mental health* (pp. 95–127). Cham: Springer International Publishing.

Hook, D. (2007). *Foucault, psychology and the analytics of power*. London: Palgrave Macmillan.

Horwitz, A. V., & Wakefield, J. C. (2007). *The loss of sadness: How psychiatry transformed normal sorrow into depressive disorder*. New York: Oxford University Press.

Horwitz, A. V., & Wakefield, J. C. (2012). *All we have to fear: Psychiatry's transformation of natural anxieties into medical disorders*. New York: Oxford University Press.

House, R. (2004). *Therapy beyond modernity: Deconstructing and transcending profession-centred therapy*. London: Karnac.

House, R. (2010). *In, against and beyond therapy: Critical essays toward a "post-professional" era*. Ross-on-Wye: PCCS Books.

Huxley, A. (1932). *Brave new world*. New York: Harper & Brothers.

Illich, I. (1977). *Limits to medicine: Medical nemesis: The expropriation of health*. Harmondsworth: Penguin.

Illouz, E. (2003). *Oprah Winfrey and the glamour of misery: An essay on popular culture*. New York: Columbia University Press.
Illouz, E. (2007). *Cold intimacies: The making of emotional capitalism*. Cambridge: Polity Press.
Illouz, E. (2008). *Saving the modern soul: Therapy, emotions, and the culture of self-help*. Berkeley: University of California Press.
Ingleby, D. (Ed.). (1980). *Critical psychiatry: The politics of mental health*. New York: Pantheon Books.
Jorm, A. F. (2000). Mental health literacy: Public knowledge and beliefs about mental disorders. *British Journal of Psychiatry, 177*(5), 396–401.
Keohane, K., & Petersen, A. (Eds.). (2013). *The social pathologies of contemporary civilization*. New York: Routledge.
Kramer, P. D. (1997). *Listening to prozac: A psychiatrist explores antidepressant drugs and the remaking of the self*. New York: Penguin Books.
Krans, B. (2016, May 9). The 17 best depression blogs of 2016. Accessed November 28, 2016, from http://www.healthline.com/health/depression/best-blogs-of-the-year#3.
Lakoff, A. (2005). *Pharmaceutical reason: Knowledge and value in global psychiatry*. Cambridge: Cambridge University Press.
Layard, R. (2005). *Happiness: Lessons from a new science*. London: Penguin.
Lazzarato, M. (2014). *Signs and machines: Capitalism and the production of capitalism*. Semiotext(e): Los Angeles.
Lunau, K. (2012). The mental health crisis on campus. Accessed November 30, 2016, from http://www.macleans.ca/education/uniandcollege/the-mental-health-crisis-on-campus/.
Martin, J., & McLellan, A. (2013). *The education of selves: How psychology transformed students*. New York: Oxford University Press.
McLaughlin, K. (2012). *Surviving identity: Vulnerability and the psychology of recognition*. London: Routledge.
Miller, P., & Rose, N. (2008). *Governing the present: Administering economic, social and personal life*. Cambridge: Polity Press.
Moncrieff, J. (2008). *The myth of the chemical cure: A critique of psychiatric drug treatment*. New York: Palgrave MacMillan.
Monk, G., Winslade, J., & Sinclair, S. (2008). *New horizons in multicultural counseling*. Thousand Oaks, CA: Sage.
Morey, M. E., Arora, P., & Stark, K. D. (2015). Multiple-stage screening of youth depression in schools. *Psychology in the Schools, 52*(8), 800–814.
Morozov, E. (2013). *To save everything, click here: The folly of technological solutionism*. New York: PublicAffairs.

Moses, I. (2000). Is it ethical to deceive managed care companies? A panel of the new editors of the journal of contemporary psychotherapy. *Journal of Contemporary Psychotherapy, 30*(3), 217–237.

Moss, P., & Teghtsoonian, K. (2008). *Contesting illness: Processes and practices.* Toronto: University of Toronto Press.

Murgia, M. (2016, June 21). Dr google will see you now: New health symptom checker takes on GPs. *The telegraph*. Accessed November 28, 2016, from http://www.telegraph.co.uk/technology/2016/06/21/dr-google-will-see-you-now-new-health-symptom-checker-takes-on-g/.

Nesi, J., & Prinstein, M. J. (2015). Using social media for social comparison and feedback-seeking: Gender and popularity moderate associations with depressive symptoms. *Journal of Abnormal Child Psychology, 43*(8), 1427–1438.

Newnes, C. (2011). Toxic psychology. In M. Rapley, J. Moncrieff, & J. Dillon (Eds.), *De-medicalizing misery: Psychiatry, psychology and the human condition* (pp. 211–225). New York: Palgrave Macmillan.

Parikh, S. V. (2015). Improving access to psychosocial treatments: Integrating patient, provider, and systems approaches. *Canadian Journal of Psychiatry, 60*(6), 242–244.

Parker, I. (Ed.). (2015). *Handbook of critical psychology*. New York: Routledge.

Peale, N. V. (1952). *The power of positive thinking and the amazing results of positive thinking*. New York: Prentice Hall.

Perls, F. S. (1969). *Gestalt therapy verbatim*. Gouldsboro: The Gestalt Journal Press.

Pinder, C. C., & Bourgeois, V. W. (1982). Controlling tropes in administrative science. *Administrative Science Quarterly, 27*(4), 641.

Prilleltensky, I. (1994). *The morals and politics of psychology: Psychological discourse and the status quo*. Albany: State University of New York Press.

Prince, M. J. (2008). Claiming a disability benefit as contesting social citizenship. In P. Moss & K. Teghtsoonian (Eds.), *Contesting illness: Processes and practice* (pp. 28–46). Toronto: University of Toronto Press.

Ravenscroft, I. (2016, August 16). Folk psychology as theory. *Stanford encyclopedia of philosophy*. Accessed November 28, 2016, from http://plato.stanford.edu/entries/folkpsych-theory/.

Rich, E., & Miah, A. (2017). Mobile, wearable and ingestible health technologies: Towards a critical research agenda. *Health Sociology Review, 26*(1), 84–97.

Richards, G. (2010). *Putting psychology in its place: Critical historical perspectives* (3rd ed.). New York: Routledge.

Rose, N. (1990). *Governing the soul: The shaping of the private self*. New York: Routledge.

Rose, N. (1997). *Inventing our selves: Psychology, power, and personhood*. Cambridge: Cambridge University Press.

Rosenbaum, P. J., & Liebert, H. (2015). Reframing the conversation on college student mental health. *Journal of College Student Psychotherapy, 29*(3), 179–196.

Sampson, E. E. (1981). Cognitive psychology as ideology. *American Psychologist, 36*(7), 730–743.

Scheff, T. J. (1967). *Mental illness and social processes*. New York: Harper & Row.

Seligman, L. (2004). *Diagnosis and treatment planning in counseling* (3rd ed.). New York: Springer.

Sennett, R. (1981). *Authority*. New York: Vintage.

Sflakidou, S., & Kefalopoulou, M. (2015). The person-centred approach as an ideological discourse: A discourse analysis of person-centred counsellors' accounts on their way of being. *European Journal of Psychotherapy & Counselling, 17*(2), 179.

Shorter, E. (1992). *From paralysis to fatigue: A history of psychosomatic illness in the modern era*. New York: Free Press.

Shorter, E. (2013). *How everyone became depressed: The rise and fall of the nervous breakdown*. Oxford: Oxford University Press.

Smith, A. J., & Siegel, R. F. (1985). Feminist therapy: Redefining power for the powerless. In L. E. A. Walker & L. B. Rosewater (Eds.), *Handbook of feminist therapy: Women's issues in psychotherapy* (pp. 13–21). New York: Springer.

Starker, S. (2002). *Oracle at the supermarket: The American preoccupation with self-help books*. New Brunswick: Transaction Publishers.

Steers, M. N., Wickham, R. E., & Acitelli, L. K. (2014). Seeing everyone else's highlight reels: How facebook usage is linked to depressive symptoms. *Journal of Social and Clinical Psychology, 33*(8), 701–731.

Steiner, C. (2012). *Automate this: How algorithms came to rule our world*. New York: Penguin.

Stewart, D. W., Walker, J. R., Beatie, B., Reynolds, K. A., Hahlweg, K., Leonhart, M., et al. (2014). Postsecondary students' information needs and pathways for help with stress, anxiety, and depression/Les besoins d'information des étudiants postsecondaires et les parcours conçus pour réduire le stress, l'anxiété, et la dépression. *Canadian Journal of Counselling and Psychotherapy (Online), 48*(3), 356–374.

Strong, T., Ross, K. H., & Sesma-Vazquez, M. (2015). Counselling the (self?) diagnosed client: Generative and reflective conversations. *British Journal of Guidance and Counselling, 43*(5), 598–610.

Taylor, C. (1985). *Human agency and language: Philosophical papers 1*. Cambridge: Cambridge University Press.

Taylor, C. (1989). *Sources of the self: The making of the modern identity*. Cambridge, MA: Harvard University Press.

Taylor, C. (1997). *Philosophical arguments*. Cambridge, MA: Harvard University Press.

Thompson, R. (2012). Screwed up, but working on it: (Dis)ordering the self through e-stories. *Narrative Inquiry, 22*(1), 86–104.

Toscano, A., & Kinkle, J. (2015). *Cartographies of the absolute: An aesthetics of the economy for the twenty-first century*. London: Zero Books.

TRC (Truth and Reconciliation Commission of Canada). (2015). TRC findings. Accessed November 28, 2016, from http://www.trc.ca/websites/trcinstitution/index.php?p=890.

Walters, W. (2012). *Governmentality: Critical encounters*. New York: Routledge.

Whitaker, R. (2010). *Anatomy of an epidemic: Magic bullets, psychiatric drugs and the astonishing rise of mental illness*. New York: Broadway Paperbacks.

WHO (World Health Organization). (2003). WHO definition of health. Accessed November 28, 2016, from http://www.who.int/about/definition/en/print.html.

Wylie, M. S. (1995). Diagnosing for dollars? *Family Therapy Networker, 19*(3), 22–23.

6

Medicating and Technologizing Our Diagnosable Lives

> What is truly threatening to psychiatry is evidence that both the *form and content* of emotional distress and "disordered" behavior are *systematically, meaningfully and inseparably related* to social context and life experience.
> (Boyle 2011: 35, emphasis in original)

Mental health, to the public, has increasingly and understandably become like any other aspect of health; if there are concerns, there are correct professional diagnoses to be made and science-backed medical treatments to be prescribed. The prevalence of this understanding grew with the prevalence of mental and substance abuse disorders which have now surpassed stroke, diabetes, and HIV as the leading causes of non-fatal illnesses worldwide (Whiteford et al. 2013). With so much media attention on mental health and illness, prospective patients are effectively recruited to monitor symptoms and consult doctors for particular medications (Busfield 2010), as rates for diagnosable mental disorders have accelerated (Angell 2011). The impetus for this rise, suggest some critics, has been a brain-based chemical imbalance "myth," which has been widely taken up by professionals as well as the clients/patients they serve (e.g. Deacon 2013). Mythical or real, medications are intended

T. Strong, *Medicalizing Counselling*, Palgrave Studies in the Theory and History of Psychology, DOI 10.1007/978-3-319-56699-3_6

to provide symptom relief, and some looking into their use for mental health concerns see either an "epidemic" (Whitaker 2010) or at least a concerning upward trend, particularly for depression (Mojtabai and Olfson 2013). As DSM-IV editor and DSM-5 critic, Allen Frances (2013: 28), suggested, "The business model of the pharmaceutical industry depends on extending the realm of illness." What this extension means for counselling is the focus of this chapter, as the exposés on "Big Pharma" and mental health can be found elsewhere (e.g. Healy 2012; Whitaker and Cosgrove 2015).

Central to our considerations in this chapter will be how medications, and new forms of technology, may be shaping counselling's intersection (or conflation) with contemporary mental health services. How does the conversational work of counselling fit within a mental health landscape that turned heavily biomedical (i.e. focused on prescription medications) after the introduction of the DSM-III and EBP, and in a landscape anticipating further diagnostic developments (see Goldfried 2013, 2016)? This is a chapter that also explores further a developing frontier of new mental health technologies based on medical and neuroscience developments (Huguet et al. 2016; Milev et al. 2016). The heuristic guiding this chapter is: what role does counselling have in an increasingly medicalized world where medications and technologies may be adjunctive to counselling, or vice versa?

Mood-Altering Substances and Counselling?

Psychoactive substances have always been part of Shamanistic traditions of practice some associate with counselling (Harner 1990; Krippner 2002). Freud (1885) himself experimented with prescribing the use of cocaine for its healing potentials. However, it was not until the years after the Second World War that medications for anxiety (Tone 2008) and depression (Greenberg 2010) began to expand into the ambiguous zone psychoanalysts had deemed "neurotic." In Greenberg's colorful language, this was an era in which "depression doctors turned away from biography and back to biology" (2010: 126).

Freud's cross-over from his start in neurology to conversationally focused psychoanalysis (see Jones 1974) is frequently touted as modern counselling's starting place. The return back to biology was enabled by etiology-agnostic DSM-III diagnoses; what mattered was what alleviated symptomatic suffering. While medications like Thorazine and lithium became part of the still-counselling psychiatrist's mid-twentieth-century pharmacopeia for more serious, psychotic kinds of mental disorders (schizophrenia, bipolar disorder) (Whitaker 2010), depression and anxiety medications were usually targeted for use by general practitioners. These new medications for milder "disorders" inaugurated a new, and less conversationally focused "journey into the economy of melancholy," as Greenberg entitled another article (2007).

While alcohol has been recognized as a form of self-medication for depression or anxiety for centuries (Valverde 1998), and recreational drugs provided related forms of escape for millennia (Taylor 1966), pharmaceutical companies have only relatively recently addressed human miseries. Any discussion of medications or "drugs" invariably requires some consideration of potential abuse or addictive effects (e.g. Booth 1997), but that will not be the focus here. Instead, my interest shall be with how counselling and prescription medication use—most notably use of antidepressants and anti-anxiolytic medications—find potential overlaps, extending to how counselling is influenced by those overlaps. The depressions and anxieties of interest here will be "sub-clinical," so as to skirt obvious issues associated with severely debilitating depression or anxiety (see Horwitz and Wakefield 2007, 2012, respectively). Our primary focus will remain the "worried well" or "mildly melancholic" potential clients who come to counselling with normal life difficulties (Aubrey 1983; Hahn 1955) or Szasz's (1961) "problems in living."

In a popularized *New York Times* sketch of the history of medication for depression, Mukherjee (2012) cited a serendipitous discovery that occurred in a sanatorium treating tubercular patients in the early 1950s. That discovery—iproniazid—had an observed effect on patients' moods and behaviors and prompted consideration of how the same effects might be generalizable to other people affected by disturbances of moods and behaviors—or "depressed brains" (Mukherjee 2012).

Prior to this time, opioids and amphetamines were used to respond to depressive symptoms (Weber and Emrich 1988). Between the time of iproniazid's discovery, and the eventual articulation of the neurotransmitter hypothesis (Siever and Davis 1985) that came to inform the development of Prozac, the market for antidepressants was relatively small and focused on the use of "tricyclics" and tranquilizers like valium (Greenberg 2010).

While some researchers clearly wanted to keep symptomatic concerns like depression and anxiety at least partly nested in sociocultural context (Engel 1977), increasingly the cultural and medical focus was turning to the brain. Introduced in the 1980s, Prozac, Paxil, and Zoloft ushered in a new era for medicating the symptoms Greenberg (2013) has referred to as human "woe." Central to this era's thinking on depression and anxiety were metaphors of failing neurotransmitters or broken brains that transformed the prescribing patterns of physicians and psychiatrists (Abramson 2004; Kirsch 2009). Marketer-in-chief for this thinking was psychiatrist Peter Kramer (1997) whose *Listening to Prozac* made the case for antidepressants as personality enhancers. For Kramer, there had been a too-accepted low or bottom to people's emotional and cognitive experiences that could be elevated with medications like Prozac. Problems in one's thinking and feelings could also be pharmaceutically *managed* differently, the premise being that such problems were brain-based. An illustration of this premise comes from Lauren Slater's *Prozac Diary*: "Behind every crooked thought … lies a crooked molecule" (1998: 108). A new brain-based, antidepressant-enabling kind of biopower was being made possible: refashioning or repurposing one's mental health biology (Fraser 2001; Fullagar 2009).

In 1990, the first President Bush announced "the decade of the Brain," launching neuroscience into what seemed like a promising era (Jones and Mendell 1999). Brain damage—whether from strokes, injuries, Alzheimer, and so on—became a target for new treatments, and seemed prone to what some critics have referred to "ontological gerrymandering" (Woolgar and Pawluch 1985). Such gerrymandering occurs when explanations are extended into new and questionable realms. The brain-based, neurotransmitter-deficit model of mood disorders widely circulating in the public consciousness, along with aggressive marketing of mood-enhancing medications, ushered in a new kind of politics (Rose 2001). No longer was biology our destiny—an affective and physiological transformability was seen to be enabled by medications that could alter unwanted moods, and even overcome sexual impotency (Fishman 2010). With respect to brains and moods, whether one wanted to attribute these to life circumstances or serotonin issues, for many it didn't matter; there were new pharmaceutical ways to manage our quality of living.

Did it matter that brain-based and pharmaceutically responsive understandings of human concerns could trump understandings associated with Szasz's (1961) "problems in living"? The short answer of psychiatric historian Edward Shorter (1998), when contrasting Prozac and Freud for their effectiveness in addressing depression, was: no. This historical assessment came despite some psychiatrists earlier suggesting people talk "back to Prozac" (Breggin and Breggin 1994). It may seem I am singling out Prozac, when the issues I raise translate far beyond the effects a particular medication might have on one's well-being or on counselling. My concern is with how the brain-based view that coincided with a rise in the use of antidepressants and anti-anxiolytic medications competed for, and came to prominently feature in, the public's imagination (see Taylor 2004) . This brain-based view of human concerns is hardly restricted to medication use, but a cultural dialogue was emerging between pharmaceutical companies, prescribing professionals, and people for whom medications were a means to minimize misery.

A particular kind of logic was on the rise among those in the pharmaceutical industry; that perhaps the key to minimizing symptoms and optimizing emotional and cognitive functioning was attainable through a reversal of the normal diagnose-and-treat logic associated with medicalization. While an initial DSM diagnosis might start a medication process, the true diagnosis and treatment would be based on patients' responsiveness to medications, in what Lakoff (2005) referred to as "pharmaceutical reasoning." This kind of reasoning seems counterintuitive and for good reason. Recall that the DSM-III and its successors were developed on the basis of identifying, carefully describing, and classifying symptom clusters (Frances 2013). Unlike other disorders of health, the causal or etiological mechanisms behind such diagnosable clusters, or disorders, were still unknown. Whether mood-related concerns of the kind that many, like Kramer (1997), in the 1990s saw as brain-based were in fact thus based has been a contentious source of debate (see Healy 2004; Kirsch 2009). Lakoff's description of pharmaceutical reasoning suggests an industry premise that many would find troubling: that every person can be optimally pharmaceutically *managed*, and the means for doing so involves "truing" up one's responsiveness to customized prescription regimens. While such reasoning can seem sinister and over the top, people have purportedly been reconstructing personal identities in light of what medication use can enable (e.g. Hewitt et al. 2000). While some see disease-mongering coming from the pharmaceutical companies (Moynihan et al. 2002) others see new forms of biopower (Fraser 2001; Maher 2008).

Pharmaceuticalization?

Questions have been raised by Abraham (2010) as to whether "pharmaceuticalization" can be properly seen as an aspect of what medicalization enables, or if it merits study as its own sociological phenomenon. Williams and colleagues (2009: 37) have defined pharmaceuticalization as transforming "human conditions, capacities or capabilities into pharmaceutical matters of treatment or enhancement." Pharmaceuticalization is perhaps best understood as a logic developed to sell quality of life to consumers on a basis that McCormack (2007) referred to as "molecular affect." Molecular affect will be a struggle for those who like to philosophically separate the notions of spirit and matter, since drugs, it would seem, operate in a kind of middle zone, modulating our spirits through the material effects of pharmaceutical interventions. From a commercial standpoint, pharmaceuticalization is like any other trend in the global economy, and that means seeking new markets, lobbying governments, and finding new ways to manage or enhance one's moods (Moynihan and Cassels 2005; Relman and Angell 2002; Watters 2010), or rebranding those unwanted moods for pharmaceutical purposes (see Horwitz 2010).

For those who lived through the 1960s, the notion of mood enhancement is reminiscent of a phrase from that era's recreational drug culture "better living through the chemistry," with a contemporary version being the growth of "cognitive enhancement" drugs (Coveney et al. 2011). For Abraham (2010) and others (e.g. Rapley et al. 2011; Rose 2006), however, the greatest concerns arise from how the marketing and science arms of the pharmaceutical industry converge in an expansionary way. Economic success can be measured through evidence of increasing patient advocacy for new medications, and from physician responses to incentive schemes to prescribe new medications (see Applbaum 2006; or Bell and Figert 2012). Greenberg (2013) offers an interesting and critical perspective on what such pharmaceuticalizing means for the worried well, having himself been a patient, a therapist, and a participant in research trials for new medications. A clear upshot of pharmaceuticalization is a more symptom and drug-savvy consuming public (Hotze et al. 2011; Lakoff 2008). Symptom monitoring and patient advocacy (by individuals and self-help groups) suggests a view that is consistent with the pharmaceutical reasoning developed in Chap. 5 in the quality of our emotional lives is to be disciplined and managed, with medications central to those efforts (Padamsee 2011).

For some time, there has been a debate over the relative effectiveness of counselling approaches when considered or comparatively evaluated with medication use (Bandelow et al. 2015; Guidi et al. 2016), or when combined (i.e. medication and counselling; Busch and Sandberg 2016; Dalrymple 2015; Rush et al. 1977). Counselling makes therapeutic differences, but questions arise when counselling is comparatively evaluated with prescription medication trials: over the enduring effectiveness of one over the other, over how to combine medications and therapy, and over the relative costs and professionals' time involved (Busch and Sandberg 2016). While some evidence suggests an increase in counselling by psychiatrists has been occurring (e.g. Hadjipavlou et al. 2015), the jury remains out on the counselling versus antidepressant treatment debate (e.g. Cuijpers et al. 2014b).

While the debate persists, some psychologists (e.g. Ax et al. 2008) have advocated for prescribing privileges across different jurisdictions, to play a more central role in mental health service provision (Melchert 2011). Counsellors have tended to view this debate from a training and literacy perspective, seeing it as important to know the medications clients take, so they can work more effectively with health-care professionals involved in their clients' treatment (Kaut and Dickinson 2007; Schaefer and Wong-Wylie 2008). Some see medication use as an example of client agency that can be integrated within meaning- and strengths-focused counselling approaches (Griffith and Griffith 1994). While research into counselling approaches and specific counselling interventions consistently shows that counselling is helpful (Wampold and Imel 2015), the science behind such evaluations continues to be questioned. For example, a recent pilot study indicated that person-centered and CBT counselling approaches can help patients with sub-clinical levels of depression (Freire et al. 2015), while a meta-analysis of supportive and non-directive counselling approaches for depression suggested such approaches made effective differences in clients' lives (Cuijpers et al. 2012). Some counsellors, after reviews of the medication effectiveness literature for common counselling concerns, have taken strong ethical stands that medications are not an effective long-term solution (e.g. Sparks 2016). Regardless, on the comparative effectiveness of medication versus therapy, current consensus seems to favor a combination of both medications and counselling (Cuijpers et al. 2014a).

Very different logics of care can become relevant to or salient in the conversations counsellors hope to have with clients (see Mol 2008). For Mol, it comes down to priorities based on marketplace economics (i.e. a logic of choice) or relational responsibility (logic of care), and pharmaceuticalization and other developments play out into the former logic. A needless binary can emerge over what causes therapeutic change, or what role clients' agentive efforts make with respect to desired change, though counsellors don't necessarily have to take sides (see Battistella et al. 2003). This said, such agency (pill vs client) can still be difficult to sort out and counsellors can feel, as Craig Newnes (2011) suggested, that they are peripheral to a pharmaceutically dominated world where, in clients' eyes, mental health's real work is done.

Brain-Based Developments

Developments in neuroscience have only accelerated the medicalizing and pharmaceuticalizing process I have been describing. Whether seen as a new means to monitor changes to one's emotional well-being and personality (Dumit 2004), to inform interventions targeting the brain's "neuroplasticity" (e.g. Beaudoin 2014), or to account for the quality of one's relationships (Siegel 2012), neuroscience has become an authoritative, current discourse of human subjectivity (Stam 2015). As mentioned in Chap. 3, the NIMH removed research funding for DSM-5-based diagnosed disorders and treatment, and shifted to a neuroscience-based approach to diagnosis and researching interventions informed by Research Domain Criteria (Insel 2013; Insel et al. 2010). This direction reflects a view that the best evidence of disorders is neurobiological, a move that helps to sidestep the former centrality of patient self-report in diagnosing and monitoring patient concerns. As Kirmayer and Crafa (2014) indicated, it is a shift that is somewhat misplaced for overlooking the social components of "psychopathology," including those components associated with practitioner–patient interaction. However, neuroscience evidence does provide a means to both standardize and personalize one's medical interventions based on tracking such things as personal responses to medication (Gordon et al. 2005).

There are some aspects of neuroscience which are seen to provide more optimism than a medication-managed direction; discussed in Chap. 3 as pharmaceutical reasoning. The brain's "neuroplasticity"—its modifiability in response to cognitive and other forms of intervention—has become central to therapists and educators who have taken up a neuroscience-informed approach to their practice (Beaudoin 2014; Cozolino 2010; Doidge 2015). This is a use of neuroscience that can be best understood in terms of evidence that shows correspondences with, and changes in, particular aspects of brain functioning (Dumit 2004). There is, however, a curious way in which brain functioning sometimes gets discussed that is germane to our reflections here, and that is the centrality sometimes given to brain processes or regions of the brain. The notion that my frontal lobes "executively" organized this year's successful Christmas party would be an example of what some call a "mereological fallacy" (Bennett et al. 2007). This fallacy highlights how brain parts, like other body parts, are not the agents of origins of our actions; that would be like saying my knees took me out for a walk. Nor are our brains machines, despite repeated efforts to reduce them to such a metaphor, however highly functioning they might be regarded as computational devices (Pinker 1999).

Neuroscience, like pharmaceuticalization, has, for its therapeutic focus, tended to steer humans away from the circumstances and preferences in their lives, to inwardly compel attention to aspects of one's biological functioning that are mostly understood to be beyond their influence to understand differently or alter (Dingwall et al. 2003). Both convey a medicalizing sense that the quality of human life—not uncommonly—is best approached and managed in ways that subordinate human agency to make us patients. A different kind of personhood or clienthood than that discussed in previous chapters begins to emerge through a new form of subjectification based on new kinds of objective science. In the language of Rose and Abi-Rached (2013: 140): "At root, the neurobiological project in psychiatry finds its limit in the simple and often repeated fact: mental disorders are problems of persons, not of brains."

What neuroscience and pharmaceutical developments mean for the conversational work of counselling is a matter of potential debate. When the functioning of people's synapses or brain parts focus cultural concern or expected intervention, the relevance of counselling can be called into question. Concern has been expressed that with, such a focus, needs for a pharmaceutically oriented psychiatry only grow, while social justice efforts, services to marginalized peoples, and needs for honoring cultural diversity become further obscured and subordinated (see Burstow et al. 2014). Some critics see potentials for psychiatric oppression, as Pitts–Taylor (2016: 6) highlights: "reduction of social problems to neurobiology can also result in the subjection of individuals and groups to techniques of neurogovernance." The natural question some might ask is who will be doing this kind of "neuro-governing"?

As with other psychology and mental health developments, potential new forms of agency may be enabled by neuroscience, while others see a further surrender of personal autonomy to mental health professionals. For example, the brain's neuroplasticity enables a kind of "neuronal self" that is well suited to marketplace requirements for self-agentive entrepreneurialism (Pitts-Taylor 2010). Others see new understandings, therapeutic approaches, and forms of collaboration arising from interpersonal neurobiological knowledge (see Siegel 2012). Neuroscience continues to promise new possibilities, while a half-century of pharmaceutical science into mental health treatments may have stalled, with some larger pharmaceutical companies moving on to more profitable investments (Miller 2010). The hoped-for intersection of neuroscience with new psychiatric medications has not transpired (Hyman 2014), though some are optimistic about what counselling might offer based on new neuroscience theorizing (LeDoux and Pine 2016).

Where the pharmaceutical world and the neuroscience world have been converging is around a cultural development that melds scientific knowledge and its applications—to enable risk management (Beck 1992; Dumit 2012; Hogarth 2015). This was part of the customizing process referred to when discussing Lakoff's (2005) "pharmaceutical reasoning," and relates to the enhancement potentials afforded by new medications and technologies. This is the logic that suggests that our mental health is an ongoing management issue; one requiring use of what Hook (2007), following Foucault, calls "affective technologies of the self." On one hand, there are more ways to manage chronic disruptions to mood and performance, for concerns that seemingly can't be overcome (Dumit 2012; Quintero and Nichter 2011). One can become a "pharmaceutical person," in Emily Martin's (2006) parlance, someone engaged in minimizing symptoms and optimizing in pharmaceutical benefits, through mitigating unwanted side effects that can come from living a pharmaceutically managed life. On the other hand, people increasingly approach emotional well-being as others have approached fitness and nutrition—for example, by designing, disciplining, and optimizing their resilience and emotional intelligence (Algoe and Fredrickson 2011). How counsellors' efforts to be helpful fit within these self-management regimes can become another source of tension with such medicalized or pharmaceuticalized developments. What role will counsellors have when the affects and intellects of clients are understood to be rendered self-designable and self-manageable by pharmaceutical and technological means?

Mental Health Technologies?

Such new ways of fashioning personal well-being and managing disruptions to it have become a frontier of sorts, for pharmaceutical as well as technological developments. While electro-convulsive therapies seem seldom used these days, a slightly different and more targeted version has emerged that draws on insights from neuroscience, to enable "neurostimulation" of cognitive abilities (Dubljević 2015; Farah et al. 2004). It is a technology that, for some readers, may seem lifted from the writing of cyberpunk author, William Gibson (1984), and it is a technology that has been outstripping ethical developments associated with its use (Dubljević 2015; Farah 2012). The simple version of it is as a kind of neural, transcranial massage that can boost atrophied areas of cognitive functioning, but it also is stimulation being used to generally enhance mood and cognitive performance. Google © cites a US patent (U.S. Patent No. US9155891 B2 2015) for a "Current management system for a stimulation output stage of an implantable neurostimulation system." This kind of stimulation should not seem too much a stretch if one considers other such health-management resources as cardiac pacemakers, or even hearing aids. Guidelines for therapeutic use or evaluative research of neurostimulation are still in their infancy (Cimpianu et al. 2016; Milev et al. 2016), though the recurring message is that neurostimulation is a promising new technology for addressing mood disorders and other mental health concerns.

The commercial and corporate world is well ahead in making use of developments from mental health research and treatment. As William Davies (2015) highlighted in a recent and provocative book, *The Happiness Industry*, the methods as well as the knowledge from neuroscience and mental health research have enabled many breakthroughs in terms of business applications for enhancing our well-being. Davies cites one striking example: specially designed blankets with sensors that show flight attendants when our moods might benefit from their intervention. Davies' concern partly relates to the assumptions brought to these new technologies for well-being, big data kinds of assumptions that position users of such technology to more fully participate in the marketplace. As technology and media critic Wendy Chun (2016, Kindle Location 773) has written: "The media have imploded in the social. YOU are a character in a drama called Big Data" (emphasis in original). There is a sense in which a big data approach can enable people to program their technologies (e.g. neurostimulation) according to the norms of their personal behavior and functioning, to live according to those norms. But, extending this sense, Chun sees disruptions to our programmed normality requiring resets of our technology-enabled lives according to the following formula: habit + crisis = update. Updates would be based on solutions already developed for us by artificial intelligence (AI) (Morozov 2013).

Such new mood-shaping, norm-based technologies pose challenging questions regarding personal autonomy and programming. Specifically, concerns can arise about where and how the "self-agency" of people making use of such technologies finds a serendipitous confluence with consumerism (Illouz 2007; Lazzarato 2011). Such limiting forms of self-agency see people adapting to environments they can decreasingly influence. In Marxist terms, such affective and marketplace forms of technology-enabled self-agency exemplify a kind of "false consciousness" (Eagleton 1991), an ideology-fostered illusion of how to best exercise our personal freedom given how things are. The ideology is neoliberalism and the technologies can be seen to optimize our participation and consumption in life's marketplace (Harvey 2005; Monbiot 2016).

These last words may remind readers of longstanding concerns critics have had about counsellors supporting clients to adapt to unjust experiences (Ingleby 1980; Rose 1990). A current version of these concerns can similarly challenge some counsellors: that psychology and the approaches to counselling enabled by it, are complicit in enabling a neoliberal "self-governance" (Ferraro 2016; Loewenthal 2015; Triliva and Georga 2014). Such self-governance tends to be focused on succeeding, however marginally, in a highly competitive economy (Standing 2011). An example of this concern has been playing out in the UK where the government's recently mandated "get to work therapy" (to enable "workfare") was countered by a growing group of counsellors who see this as an unethical abuse of the economically disadvantaged (*The Guardian* 2015). While counsellors may object to expectations they "serve" the public in such ways, the perennial challenge is with helping clients cope with harsh realities. Drugs and technologies provide means to cope with such unwanted circumstances. Dystopian science fiction novels, like Gibson's (1984) *Neuromancer*, are partly premised on the notion that reality is unalterable, making technological and pharmaceutical escapes from it logical. Chun's (2016) review of recent and forecasted technologies raises questions about where and how technology might help counselling clients cope, or what "update" their technologies or lives might require.

There is a component of what I have been raising that relates to a particular view of science and life that Davies (2015) takes to task in his *Happiness Industry*. This is a view Davies refers to as "Benthamite," based on the empiricist ideas of the nineteenth-century philosopher, Jeremy Bentham. It is also a view that suggests that the correlates of our happiness (or, for our purposes, mental health) can be objectively known, quantified, and engineered to produce desired results. This, as things turn out, is also the view taken by many in the field of AI, the field that produces the smart devices, apps, and technologies we have been discussing (Chun 2011, 2016). AI is partly developed according to the premise that normative knowledge can be objectively formalized and then used as the basis for decisions humans might otherwise have to make themselves. At the level of one's personal behavior, a simplified version of this would be that, because eight times out of ten one will do something in a circumstance, this objectified predictability enables technology to make such decisions "on one's behalf" in that circumstance. This is how Amazon can make "acceptable" purchase suggestions to me. AI takes a Benthamite and normative view of human experience, and our technologies tend to be based on this view.

For decades, philosopher Hubert Dreyfus (1967, 2013) has been suggesting that AI and the computers it enables can never fully imitate or emulate humans because computers lack bodies, and with them desires, needs, and other human attributes. Human knowledge and formalized computer knowledge (AI) are different, because, unlike AI, human knowledge is not static or general—it is always used in embodied and situated activities and engagements (Dreyfus and Dreyfus 1986). He does not see such engagements and activities as conceptually mediated, or AI programmable (Dreyfus 2013). While humans can develop formerly unbelievable technologies like driverless cars, or companion robots, to what extent can smart devices and apps address human needs associated with one's mental health, or enhance aspects of one's quality of life?

Extending the Benthamite and AI critique a bit further, psychology itself has had to grapple with the kinds of concerns raised in pursuing its status as a social science. Arguably, social science produces formalized knowledge equivalent to AI, without achieving the Benthamite ideal of truly objective knowledge. In Chap. 2 we tackled some of this when discussing discourse theory and how medicalizing discourse based on a diagnose-and-treat logic was one way of "carving nature at its joints," to coin a phrase from Plato (2005: 265d–266a). For AI aficionados, "the singularity" will soon be upon us (see Kurzweil 2005), a juncture in time where super-intelligence (Bostrom 2014) derived from AI will overtake human intelligence. But, as critics persist in saying, computers don't have motivations, intelligence, autonomy, and so on (see Searle 2014). So, the technologies developed originate from humans who use them to extend human capacities, like prosthetics they do not replace them. Why this observation matters in a review of mental health technologies relates to being smart with smart devices, to not be on an AI and technologically enabled "auto-pilot" when we need an embodied, situated response.

Long before mental health apps and smart devices were on the scene, the Benthamite wing of psychology had been hard at work seeking social science equivalents to the laws of gravity. Their version of formalized knowledge (normative and AI-like) was based on a view that experience was correctly knowable and thus controllable; a social science approach to engineering desired human outcomes. For Ken Gergen (1982), this was how social scientists were out to construct the "real and the good," as if these ever could be objectified, apart from human interpretation and values (see Taylor 1997) . That communities of social scientists—for example, behavioral psychologists—could collectively decide on such constructions and how to obtain them to the collectivity's satisfaction, is not the question here (see Latour 1987, 2005). That any social science community would claim what "real and good" should mean for the rest of us is an issue worth reflecting upon, particularly if our technologies are moving us closer to a "singularity" promising the "real and the good" that is based on that community's science.

There is yet a further aspect to this Benthamite view of psychology that is closer to home for counsellors, and it tangentially relates to what I have been calling a medicalizing discourse. Specifically, one approach to counselling (or counselling discourse) comes closer to this view, and that made it most amenable to being researched in the ways medical interventions are researched. CBT has, at different times, been proposed as a means to get more rational and perceptually objective in one's experience and conduct (see Sampson 1981). The Benthamite aspect to CBT arises in how adjudications are made of proper thinking and acting, which, admittedly, diminishing numbers of CBT-oriented counsellors today would claim as their professional prerogative (see House and Loewenthal 2008). Where contention comes up, if at all, is around "distortions" of thought—the notion that undistorted thought is about perceiving and understanding *correctly*. By extension, such distortions or maladaptive patterns of thinking are seen to negatively affect mood and behavior. The key to CBT, however, comes with evaluations of one's thinking, and in the public perception this can translate to thinking correctly, or as indicated on the public website of one America's most prestigious medical centers, the Mayo Clinic (2016): "CBT helps you become aware of *inaccurate* or negative thinking so you can view challenging situations more clearly and respond to them in a more effective way" (emphasis added). CBT was the first choice counselling approach of Lord Layard (2005; his *Happiness* prescription) and was recommended as a counselling strategy to get the unemployed to accept "workfare" (see *The Guardian* 2015). The primary reasons for such prescriptions have been related to CBT's scientific (i.e. Benthamite) backing.

Many of today's mental health apps and related technologies have adapted the psychoeducational premises of CBT (see Dellabella, n.d.). While one can find helpful resources for altering one's breathing when faced with distressing developments, such as symptom severity monitors or information from blogs, there are also apps offering guided exercises to address "distorted thoughts" (see Kaiser 2014). This focus on interventions associated with counselling approaches—that there are specific benefits associated with CBT use that make it superior—may be misguided, suggest authors of a recent and important *meta-meta*-analytic study (Wampold et al. 2017). These authors suggest turning away from specific techniques in counselling approaches and looking more broadly at the question: what makes counselling work? The consistent answer to that question has been the collaborative quality and extratherapeutic factors relevant to what the counselling relationship, and not on techniques or didactics (see Duncan et al. 2010). While our AI-enabled mental health technologies enable specific interventions, they are tools and do not negate the importance of caring relationships.

Afterthoughts on Affective Technologies

My digression into medications and technologies in this chapter has been to bring out a facet of medicalizing discourse that has become very much a part of contemporary Western culture (de Vos 2012; Illouz 2008). A technological solutionism (Morozov 2013) based on reductionist AI is popular and promises shortcuts and less odious ways of going through life. It is a solutionism that has imported the insights of social science and neuroscience, and is now wedded to technological version of medicalizing discourse focused on optimally managing or governing oneself (Rose and Abi-Rached 2013). People can embed themselves in the care promised by these technologies and medications and manage their inner worlds in ways that purportedly minimize the negative affective consequences of living in the outer world where a seemingly messier "human condition" (Arendt 1959) prevails.

Central to these reflections has been a view that society's quality of life-enhancing imagination has been competed for (see Taylor 2004) , in ways taken up by savvy consumers of mental health services and related tools that Hook (2007) referred to as "affective technologies." A different kind of citizen is being reflexively produced by these changes, as new kinds of "looping effects" (Hacking 1995) facilitate an evolving mental health culture increasingly dominated by developments in neuroscience and medicine. Self-care, as Foucault (2008) was claiming very early in our neoliberal era (Harvey 2005), would involve appropriating the knowledges and practices of psychiatry. Some of that self "care" might be seen in Furedi's (2004) "therapy culture," a growing portion of society passively enfeebled by medicalizing discourse, and too accepting of its identity implications (McLaughlin 2012). Another cultural development, however, can be seen more resourcefully, as clients take up the expert knowledge from medicalizing discourse, and apply it to themselves, and, by extension, what they request from counsellors (Strong et al. 2015) . None of this "self-agency," however, should be taken for granted, particularly when marketing campaigns (Payton and Thoits 2011) and media modelling of such ways to take care of one's mental health are so ubiquitous (Illouz 2008).

More insidious is the medicalizing message that disruptions to one's affective life can be treated, symptom-minimized, or risk-managed. Implicit in Watters' (2010) recent indictment of the effects of Western psychiatry on non-Western societies is a lament for the kinds of deskilling of longstanding cultural healing practices arising as cultures learn how to "properly" overcome newly understood mental health concerns (i.e. as DSM diagnoses). The presumption, of course, is that Western mental health science is universal, when those who study disorders cross-culturally (Bures 2016), suggest illness be understood "bioculturally." Other dimensions of care considered in this chapter have also been supplanted by today's medicalizing discourse of mental health. This can partly be seen when people took up the neurotransmitter understandings of broken brains, and the promises made but still not realized by neuroscience and new technologies based on it. Such unrealized promises illustrate the up and downsides of any discourse, pharmaceutical, neuroscience, and technological included. I prefer the optimism of scholars like Rosi Braidotti (2013), who espouses what she calls a "posthuman" view of humans agentively taking up such new cultural developments, but if she has things right a more complicated view of counselling must emerge. Regardless, the kinds of medical, neuroscientific, and technological developments we have considered leave out, like any discourse would, some very human and relational elements central to counselling, as this quote from Bures (2016) illustrates: "Computer programs, it turns out, cannot understand stories" (Kindle Location 1933).

References

Abraham, J. (2010). Pharmaceuticalization of society in context: Theoretical, empirical and health dimensions. *Sociology, 44*(4), 603–622.

Abramson, J. (2004). *Overdosed America*. New York: HarperCollins.

Algoe, S. B., & Fredrickson, B. L. (2011). Emotional fitness and the movement of affective science from lab to field. *American Psychologist, 66*(1), 35–42.

Angell, M. (2011, June 23). The epidemic of mental illness: Why? *New York Review of Books*. Accessed December 1, 2016, from http://www.nybooks.com/articles/2011/06/23/epidemic-mental-illness-why/.

Applbaum, K. (2006). Pharmaceutical marketing and the invention of the medical consumer. *PLoS Medicine, 3*(4), e189.

Aubrey, R. F. (1983). The odyssey of counseling and images of the future. *Personnel and Guidance Journal, 62*(2), 78–82.

Ax, R. K., Bigelow, B. J., Harowski, K., Meredith, J. M., Nussbaum, D., & Taylor, R. R. (2008). Prescriptive authority for psychologists and the public sector: Serving underserved health care consumers. *Psychological Services, 5*(2), 184–197.

Arendt, H. (1959). *The human condition*. Garden City, NY: Doubleday Anchor.

Braidotti, R. (2013). *The posthuman*. Cambridge: Polity Press.

Bures, F. (2016). *The geography of madness: Penis thieves, voodoo death, and the search for the meaning of the world's strangest syndromes (Kindle DX version)*. Brooklyn: Melville House.

Bostrom, N. (2014). *Superintelligence: Paths, dangers, strategies*. Oxford: Oxford University Press.

Bandelow, B., Reitt, M., Röver, C., Michaelis, S., Görlich, Y., & Wedekind, D. (2015). Efficacy of treatments for anxiety disorders: A meta-analysis. *International Clinical Psychopharmacology, 30*(4), 183–192.

Battistella, F., Bracardi, I., & Raffaelli, S. (2003). Discursive drugs: A constructivist approach to psychiatric practice. In G. Chiari & M. L. Nuzzo (Eds.),

Psychological constructivism and the social world (pp. 389–398). Milan: Franco Angeli.

Beaudoin, M.-N. (2014). *Boosting all children's social and emotional brain power: Life transforming activities*. Thousand Oaks, CA: Corwin Press.

Beck, U. (1992). *Risk society: Towards a new modernity*. London: Sage.

Bell, S. E., & Figert, A. E. (2012). Medicalization and pharmaceuticalization at the intersections: Looking backward, sideways and forward. *Social Science and Medicine, 75*(5), 775–783.

Bennett, M., Dennett, D., Hacker, P., & Searle, J. (2007). *Neuroscience and philosophy: Brain, mind, and language*. New York: Columbia University Press.

Booth, D. J. (1997). *Drugspeak: The analysis of drug discourse*. Amsterdam: Routledge.

Boyle, M. (2011). Marking the world go away, and how psychology and psychiatry benefit. In M. Rapley, J. Moncrieff, & J. Dillon (Eds.), *De-medicalizing misery: Psychiatry, psychology and the human condition* (pp. 27–43). London: Palgrave Macmillan.

Breggin, P. R., & Breggin, G. R. (1994). *Talking back to prozac: What doctors aren't telling you about today's most controversial drug*. New York: St. Martin's.

Burstow, B., LeFrançois, B. A., & Diamond, S. (2014). *Psychiatry disrupted: Theorizing resistance and crafting the (r)evolution*. Montreal: McGill-Queen's University Press.

Busch, F. N., & Sandberg, L. S. (2016). *Psychotherapy and medication: The challenge of integration*. New York: Routledge.

Busfield, J. (2010). A pill for every ill: Explaining the expansion in medicine use. *Social Science and Medicine, 70*(6), 934–941.

Chun, W. H. K. (2011). *Programmed visions: Software and memory*. Cambridge, MA: The MIT Press.

Chun, W. H. K. (2016). *Updating to remain the same: Habitual new media*. Cambridge: The MIT Press.

Cimpianu, C., Strube, W., Falkai, P., Palm, U., & Hasan, A. (2016). Vagus nerve stimulation in psychiatry: A systematic review of the available evidence. *Journal of Neural Transmission, 124,* 1–14.

Coveney, C., Gabe, J., & Williams, S. (2011). The sociology of cognitive enhancement: Medicalisation and beyond. *Health Sociology Review, 20*(4), 381–393.

Cozolino, L. (2010). *The neuroscience of psychotherapy: Healing the social brain* (2nd ed.). New York: W.W. Norton.

Cuijpers, P., Driessen, E., Hollon, S. D., et al. (2012). The efficacy of non-directive supportive therapy for adult depression: A meta-analysis. *Clinical Psychology Review, 32*(4), 280.

Cuijpers, P., Sijbrandij, M., Koole, S. L., et al. (2014a). Adding psychotherapy to antidepressant medication in depression and anxiety disorders: A meta-analysis. *World Psychiatry, 13*(1), 56–67.

Cuijpers, P., Turner, E. H., Mohr, D. C., Hofmann, S. G., Andersson, G., Berking, M., et al. (2014b). Comparison of psychotherapies for adult depression to pill placebo control groups: A meta-analysis. *Psychological Medicine, 44*(4), 685–695.

Dreyfus, H. L. (1967). Why computers must have bodies in order to be intelligent. *Review of Metaphysics, 21*(1), 13–32.

Dreyfus, H. L. (2013). The myth of the pervasiveness of the mental. In J. Schear (Ed.), *Mind, reason, and being in the world: The McDowell–Dreyfus debate* (pp. 15–40). New York: Routledge.

Dreyfus, H. L., & Dreyfus, S. E. (1986). *Mind over machine: The power of human intuition and expertise in the era of the computer*. New York: Free Press.

De Vos, J. (2012). *Psychologisation in times of globalisation*. London: Routledge.

Dellabella, H. (n.d.). *Top 10 mental health apps*. Accessed November 30, 2016, from http://www.psychiatryadvisor.com/top-10-mental-health-apps/slideshow/2608/.

Duncan, B. L., Miller, S. D., Wampold, B. E., & Hubble, M. A. (Eds.). (2010). *The heart and soul of change: Delivering what works in therapy* (2nd ed.). Washington: American Psychological Association.

Dalrymple, K. L. (2015). Combined treatments (medications plus psychotherapy). *Encyclopedia of Clinical Psychology* (pp. 1–6). Hoboken, NJ: Wiley.

Davies, W. (2015). *The happiness industry: How the government and big business sold us well-being*. London: Verso.

Deacon, B. J. (2013). The biomedical model of mental disorder: A critical analysis of its assumptions, consequences, and effects on psychotherapy research. *Clinical Psychology Review, 33*(7), 846–861.

Dingwall, R., Nerlich, B., & Hillyard, S. (2003). Biological determinism and symbolic interaction: Hereditary streams and cultural roads. *Symbolic Interaction, 26*(4), 631–644.

Doidge, N. (2015). *The brain's way of healing: Remarkable discoveries and recoveries from the frontiers of neuroplasticity*. New York: Penguin Books.

Dubljević, V. (2015). Neurostimulation devices for cognitive enhancement: Toward a comprehensive regulatory framework. *Neuroethics, 8*(2), 115–126.

Dumit, J. (2004). *Picturing personhood: Brain scans and biomedical identity.* Princeton: Princeton University Press.

Dumit, J. (2012). *Drugs for life: How pharmaceutical companies define our health.* Durham, NC: Duke University Press.

Eagleton, T. (1991). *Ideology: An introduction.* New York: Verso.

Engel, G. L. (1977). The need for a new medical model: A challenge for biomedicine. *Science, 196*(4286), 129–136.

Farah, M. J. (2012). Neuroethics: The ethical, legal, and societal impact of neuroscience. *Annual Review of Psychology, 63*(1), 571–591.

Farah, M. J., Illes, J., Cook-Deegan, R., et al. (2004). Neurocognitive enhancement: What can we do and what should we do? *Nature Review Neuroscience, 5*(5), 421–425.

Foucault, M. (2008). *History of madness.* New York: Routledge.

Furedi, F. (2004). *Therapy culture: Cultivating vulnerability in an uncertain age.* New York: Routledge.

Ferraro, D. (2016). Psychology in the age of austerity: Psychology and austerity. *Psychotherapy and Politics International, 14*(1), 17–24.

Fishman, J. R. (2010). The making of viagra. In A. E. Clarke, L. Mamo, J. R. Fosket, J. R. Fishman, & J. K. Shim (Eds.), *Biomedicalization: Technoscience, health and illness in the US* (pp. 289–306). Durham, NC: Duke University Press.

Frances, A. (2013). *Saving normal: An insider's revolt against out-of-control psychiatric diagnosis, DSM-5, big pharma, and the medicalization of ordinary life.* New York: William Morrow.

Fraser, M. (2001). The nature of prozac. *History of the Human Sciences, 14*(3), 56–84.

Freire, E., Williams, C., Messow, C., et al. (2015). Counselling versus low-intensity cognitive behavioural therapy for persistent sub-threshold and mild depression (CLICD): A pilot/feasibility randomised controlled trial. *BMC Psychiatry, 15*(1), 197.

Freud, S. (1885). On the general effects of cocaine. *Med Chir Central-Blatt, 20,* 374–375.

Fullagar, S. (2009). Negotiating the neurochemical self: Anti-depressant consumption in women's recovery from depression. *Health, 13*(4), 389–406.

Gergen, K. J. (1982). *Toward transformation in social knowledge.* New York: Springer.

Gibson, W. (1984). *Neuromancer.* New York: Ace.

Goldfried, M. R. (2013). What should we expect from psychotherapy? *Clinical Psychology Review, 33*(7), 862–869.

Goldfried, M. R. (2016). On possible consequences of national institute of mental health funding for psychotherapy research and training. *Professional Psychology: Research and Practice, 47*(1), 77–83.

Gordon, E., Cooper, N., Rennie, C., Hermens, D., & Williams, L. M. (2005). Integrative neuroscience: The role of a standardized database. *Clinical EEG and Neuroscience, 36*(2), 64–75.

Greenberg, G. (2007, May). Manufacturing depression: A journey into the economy of melancholy. *Harper's Magazine*. Accessed December 1, 2016, from http://harpers.org/archive/2007/05/manufacturing-depression/.

Greenberg, G. (2010). *Manufacturing depression: The secret history of a modern disease*. Toronto: Simon & Schuster.

Greenberg, G. (2013). *The book of woe: The DSM and the unmaking of psychiatry*. New York: Penguin.

Griffith, J., & Griffith, M. (1994). *The body speaks: Therapeutic dialogues for mind-body problems*. New York: Basic Books.

Guidi, J., Tomba, E., & Fava, G. A. (2016). The sequential integration of pharmacotherapy and psychotherapy in the treatment of major depressive disorder: A meta-analysis of the sequential model and a critical review of the literature. *American Journal of Psychiatry, 173*(2), 128–137.

House, R., & Loewenthal, D. (Eds.). (2008). *Against and for CBT: Towards a constructive dialogue*. Ross-on-Wye: PCCS Books.

Hacking, I. (1995). The looping effects of human kinds. In D. Sperber & A. J. Premack (Eds.), *Causal cognition* (pp. 351–383). Oxford: Oxford University Press.

Hadjipavlou, G., Hernandez, C. A. S., & Ogrodniczuk, J. S. (2015). Psychotherapy in contemporary psychiatric practice. *Canadian Journal of Psychiatry, 60*(6), 294–300.

Hahn, M. E. (1955). Counseling psychology. *American Psychologist, 10*(7), 279–282.

Harner, M. (1990). *The way of the shaman*. New York: Harper & Row.

Harvey, D. (2005). *A brief history of neoliberalism*. Oxford: Oxford University Press.

Healy, D. (2004). *Let them eat prozac: The unhealthy relationship between the pharmaceutical industry and depression*. New York: New York University Press.

Healy, D. (2012). *Pharmageddon*. Berkeley: University of California Press.

Hewitt, J. P., Fraser, M. R., & Berger, L. (2000). Is it me or is it prozac? Antidepressants and the construction of self. In D. Fee (Ed.), *Pathology and the postmodern: Mental illness as discourse and experience* (pp. 163–185). Thousand Oaks, CA: Sage.

Hogarth, S. (2015). Neoliberal technocracy: Explaining how and why the US food and drug administration has championed pharmacogenomics. *Social Science & Medicine (1982), 131,* 255–262.

Hook, D. (2007). *Foucault, psychology and the analytics of power*. London: Palgrave Macmillan.

Horwitz, A. V. (2010). How an age of anxiety became an age of depression. *The Milbank Quarterly, 88*(1), 112–138.

Horwitz, A. V., & Wakefield, J. C. (2007). *The loss of sadness: How psychiatry transformed normal sorrow into depressive disorder*. New York: Oxford University Press.

Horwitz, A. V., & Wakefield, J. C. (2012). *All we have to fear: Psychiatry's transformation of natural anxieties into medical disorders*. New York: Oxford University Press.

Hotze, T. D., Shah, K., Anderson, E. E., & Wynia, M. K. (2011). 'Doctor, would you prescribe a pill to help me?' A national survey of physicians on using medicine for human enhancement. *American Journal of Bioethics, 11*(1), 3–13.

Huguet, A., Rao, S., McGrath, P. J., Wozney, L., Wheaton, M., Conrod, J., et al. (2016). A systematic review of cognitive behavioral therapy and behavioral activation apps for depression. *PLoS ONE, 11*(5), e0154248.

Hyman, S. E. (2014). Revitalizing psychiatric therapeutics. *Neuropsychopharmacology, 39*(1), 220–229.

Illouz, E. (2007). *Cold intimacies: The making of emotional capitalism*. Cambridge: Polity Press.

Illouz, E. (2008). *Saving the modern soul: Therapy, emotions, and the culture of self-help*. Berkeley: University of California Press.

Ingleby, D. (Ed.). (1980). *Critical psychiatry: The politics of mental health*. New York: Pantheon Books.

Insel, T. (2013). *Post by former NIMH director Thomas Insel: Transforming diagnosis*. Accessed November 18, 2016, from https://www.nimh.nih.gov/about/directors/thomas-insel/blog/2013/transforming-diagnosis.shtml.

Insel, T., Cuthbert, B., Garvey, M., et al. (2010). Research domain criteria (RDoC): Toward a new classification framework for research on mental disorders. *American Journal of Psychiatry, 167*(7), 748–751.

Jones, E. (1974). *The life and work of Sigmund Freud*. London: Penguin Books.

Jones, E. G., & Mendell, L. M. (1999). Assessing the decade of the brain. *Science, 284*(5415), 739.

Kurzweil, R. (2005). *The singularity is near: When humans transcend biology*. New York: Penguin Books.

Kaut, K., & Dickinson, J. (2007). The mental health practitioner and psychopharmacology. *Journal of Mental Health Counseling, 29*(3), 204–225.
Kaiser, S. (2014, December 18). *Thought challenger*. Accessed December 6, 2016, from https://happinessapps.devpost.com/submissions/30931-thought-challenger.
Kirmayer, L. J., & Crafa, D. (2014). What kind of science for psychiatry? *Frontiers in Human Neuroscience, 8*, 435.
Kirsch, I. (2009). *The emperor's new drugs: Exploding the antidepressant myth*. London: Bodley Head.
Kramer, P. D. (1997). *Listening to Prozac: A psychiatrist explores antidepressant drugs and the remaking of the self.* New York: Penguin Books.
Krippner, S. C. (2002). Conflicting perspectives on shamans and shamanism: Points and counterpoints. *The American Psychologist, 57*(11), 962–978.
Latour, B. (1987). *Science in action*. Cambridge, MA: Harvard University Press.
Layard, R. (2005). *Happiness: Lessons from a new science*. London: Penguin.
Latour, B. (2005). *Reassembling the social: An introduction to actor-network-theory*. Oxford: Oxford University Press.
Lakoff, A. (2005). *Pharmaceutical reason: Knowledge and value in global psychiatry*. Cambridge: Cambridge University Press.
Lakoff, A. (2008). The right patient for the drug: Pharmaceutical circuits and the codification of illness. In E. J. Hackett, O. Amsterdamska, M. Lynch, & J. Wajcman (Eds.), *The handbook of science and technology studies* (3rd ed., pp. 741–760). Cambridge: The MIT Press.
Lazzarato, M. (2011). *The making of the indebted man: An essay on the neoliberal condition*. Semiotext(e): Los Angeles.
LeDoux, J. E., & Pine, D. S. (2016). Using neuroscience to help understand fear and anxiety: A two-system framework. *American Journal of Psychiatry, 173*(11), 1083–1093.
Loewenthal, D. (Ed.). (2015). *Critical psychotherapy, psychoanalysis and counselling: Implications for practice*. London: Palgrave Macmillan.
Mayo Clinic. (2016, February 23). *Cognitive behavioral therapy*. Accessed December 6, 2016, from http://www.mayoclinic.org/tests-procedures/cognitive-behavioral-therapy/home/ovc-20186868.
Maher, B. (2008). Poll results: Look who's doping. *Nature, 452*(7188), 674–675.
Martin, E. (2006). The pharmaceutical person. *Biosocieties, 1*(3), 273–287.
McCormack, D. P. (2007). Molecular affects in human geographies. *Environment and Planning A, 39*(2), 359–377.

McLaughlin, K. (2012). *Surviving identity: Vulnerability and the psychology of recognition*. London: Routledge.

Melchert, T. P. (2011). *Foundations of professional psychology: The end of theoretical orientations and the emergence of the biopsychosocial approach*. London: Elsevier.

Milev, R. V., Giacobbe, P., Kennedy, S. H., et al. (2016). Canadian network for mood and anxiety treatments (CANMAT) 2016 clinical guidelines for the management of adults with major depressive disorder: Section 4. neurostimulation treatments. *Canadian Journal of Psychiatry, 61*(9), 561–575.

Miller, G. (2010). Is pharma running out of brainy ideas? *Science, 329*(5991), 502–504.

Mojtabai, R., & Olfson, M. (2013). National trends in long-term use of antidepressant medications: Results from the US national health and nutrition examination survey. *Journal of Clinical Psychiatry, 75*(2), 169–177.

Mol, A. (2008). *The logic of care: Health and the problem of patient choice*. London: Routledge.

Monbiot, G. (2016, April 15). Neoliberalism: The ideology at the root of all our problems. *The Guardian*. Accessed December 27, 2016, from https://www.theguardian.com/books/2016/apr/15/neoliberalism-ideology-problem-george-monbiot.

Morozov, E. (2013). *To save everything, click here: The folly of technological solutionism*. New York: PublicAffairs.

Moynihan, R., & Cassels, A. (2005). *Selling sickness: How the world's biggest pharmaceutical companies are turning us all into patients*. New York: Nation Books.

Moynihan, R., Heath, I., & Henry, D. (2002). Selling sickness: The pharmaceutical industry and disease mongering. *British Medical Journal, 324*(7342), 886–890.

Mukherjee, S. (2012, April 19). Post-prozac nation: The science and history of treating depression. *New York Times Magazine*. Accessed December 1, 2016, from http://www.nytimes.com/2012/04/22/magazine/the-science-and-history-of-treating-depression.html.

Newnes, C. (2011). Toxic psychology. In M. Rapley, J. Moncrieff, & J. Dillon (Eds.), *De-medicalizing misery: Psychiatry, psychology and the human condition* (pp. 211–225). New York: Palgrave Macmillan.

Plato. (2005). *Phaedrus* (C. Rowe, Trans.). New York: Penguin Classics.

Padamsee, T. J. (2011). The pharmaceutical corporation and the 'good work' of managing women's bodies. *Social Science and Medicine, 72*(8), 1342–1350.

Payton, A. R., & Thoits, P. A. (2011). Medicalization, direct-to-consumer advertising, and mental illness stigma. *Society and Mental Health, 1*(1), 55–70.

Pinker, S. (1999). How the mind works. *Annals of the New York Academy of Sciences, 882*(1), 119–127.

Pitts-Taylor, V. (2010). The plastic brain: Neoliberalism and the neuronal self. *Health, 14*(6), 635–652.

Pitts-Taylor, V. (2016). *The brain's body: Neuroscience and corporeal politics.* Durham, NC: Duke University Press.

Quintero, G., & Nichter, M. (2011). Generation RX: Anthropological research on pharmaceutical enhancement, lifestyle regulation, self-medication and recreational drug use. In M. Singer & P. I. Erickson (Eds.), *A companion to medical anthropology* (pp. 339–355). Malden: Wiley.

Rapley, M., Moncrieff, J., & Dillon, J. (2011). *De-medicalizing misery: Psychiatry, psychology and the human condition.* New York: Palgrave Macmillan.

Relman, A. S., & Angell, M. (2002). America's other drug problem: How the drug industry distorts medicine and politics. *New Republic, 227*(25), 27–41.

Rose, N. (1990). *Governing the soul: The shaping of the private self.* New York: Routledge.

Rose, N. (2001). The politics of life itself. *Theory, Culture & Society, 18*(6), 1–30.

Rose, N. (2006). Disorders without borders? The expanding scope of psychiatric practice. *Biosocieties, 1*(4), 465–484.

Rose, N., & Abi-Rached, J. M. (2013). *Neuro: The new brain sciences and the management of the mind.* Princeton: Princeton University Press.

Rush, A. J., Beck, A. T., Kovacs, M., & Hollon, S. (1977). Comparative efficacy of cognitive therapy and pharmacotherapy in the treatment of depressed outpatients. *Cognitive Therapy and Research, 1*(1), 17–37.

Sampson, E. E. (1981). Cognitive psychology as ideology. *American Psychologist, 36*(7), 730–743.

Searle, J. R. (2014, October 9). What your computer can't know. *New York Review of Books*. Accessed December 6, 2016, from http://www.nybooks.com/articles/2014/10/09/what-your-computer-cant-know/.

Schaefer, D. G., & Wong-Wylie, G. (2008). Psychopharmacology training and canadian counsellors: Are we getting what we want and need? *Canadian Journal of Counselling, 42*(4), 249–261.

Shorter, E. (1998). How prozac slew Freud. *American Heritage, 49*(5). Accessed from http://www.americanheritage.com/content/how-prozac-slew-freud?page=show.

Siegel, D. J. (2012). *Pocket guide to interpersonal neurobiology: An integrative handbook of the mind.* New York: W.W. Norton.

Siever, L. J., & Davis, K. L. (1985). Overview toward a dysregulation hypothesis of depression. *American Journal of Psychiatry, 142,* 1017–1031.

Sparks, J. A. (2016). White paper: Efficacy of psychiatric drugs. *Ethical Human Psychology and Psychiatry, 18*(1), 20–28.

Stam, H. J. (2015). The neurosciences and the search for a unified psychology: The science and esthetics of a single framework. *Frontiers in Psychology, 6,* 1467.

Standing, G. (2011). *The precariat: The new dangerous class.* London: Bloomsbury.

Szasz, T. (1961). *The myth of mental illness: Foundations of a theory of personal conduct.* New York: Hoeber-Harper.

Strong, T., Ross, K. H., & Sesma-Vazquez, M. (2015). Counselling the (self?) diagnosed client: Generative and reflective conversations. *British Journal of Guidance and Counselling, 43*(5), 598–610.

Taylor, C. (1997). *Philosophical arguments.* Cambridge, MA: Harvard University Press.

The Guardian. (2015, April 17). *Austerity and a malign benefits regime are profoundly damaging mental health.* Accessed December 6, 2016, from https://www.theguardian.com/society/2015/apr/17/austerity-and-a-malign-benefits-regime-are-profoundly-damaging-mental-health.

Taylor, N. (1966). *Narcotics: Nature's dangerous gifts.* New York: Dell.

Taylor, C. (2004). *Modern social imaginaries.* Durham, NC: Duke University Press.

Tone, A. (2008). *The age of anxiety: A history of America's turbulent affair with tranquilizers.* New York: Basic Books.

Triliva, S., & Georga, A. (2014). Austerity and precarity: The social milieu creeps into the psychotherapeutic context. *Rivista di Psicologia Clinica, 1,* 140–153.

Valverde, M. (1998). *Diseases of the will: Alcohol and the dilemmas of freedom.* Cambridge: Cambridge University Press.

Wampold, B. E., & Imel, Z. E. (2015). *The great psychotherapy debate: The evidence for what makes psychotherapy work.* New York: Routledge.

Watters, E. (2010). *Crazy like us: The globalization of the American psyche.* New York: Free Press.

Weber, M. M., & Emrich, H. M. (1988). Current and historical concepts of opiate treatment in psychiatric disorders. *International Clinical Psychopharmacology, 3*(3), 255–266.

Wampold, B. E., Flückiger, C., Del Re, A. C., et al. (2017). In pursuit of truth: A critical examination of meta-analyses of cognitive behavior therapy. *Psychotherapy Research, 27*(1), 14–32.

Whitaker, R. (2010). *Anatomy of an epidemic: Magic bullets, psychiatric drugs and the astonishing rise of mental illness*. New York: Broadway Paperbacks.

Whitaker, R., & Cosgrove, L. (2015). *Psychiatry under the influence: Institutional corruption, social injury, and prescriptions for reform*. New York: Palgrave Macmillan.

Whiteford, H. A., Degenhardt, L., Rehm, J., et al. (2013). Global burden of disease attributable to mental and substance use disorders: Findings from the global burden of disease study 2010. *Lancet (London, England), 382*(9904), 1575–1586.

Williams, S. J., Seale, C., Boden, S., Lowe, P., & Lynn, D. (2009). Waking up to sleepiness. In S. Williams, J. Gabe, & P. Davis (Eds.), *Pharmaceuticals and society* (pp. 25–40). Chichester: Wiley-Blackwell.

Woolgar, S., & Pawluch, D. (1985). Ontological gerrymandering: The anatomy of social problems explanations. *Social Problems, 32*(3), 214–227.

7

Medicalizing Tensions Associated with Administering and Regulating Counselling

Is counselling for this covered by my health benefits?
(Anonymous client)

Counsellors (at least in Canada, where I and my two co-authors for this chapter, Konstantinos Chondros and Vanessa Vegter, are from) have indicated that they practice using heterogeneous (i.e. pluralistic) approaches (Gazzola et al. 2010; Strong et al. 2012). This heterogeneity can be seen as a virtue, particularly as ethical practice expands to encompass previously unaddressed dimensions of human concern (social justice, cultural inclusivity). While there may be hundreds of counselling approaches, a smaller plurality of approaches is taught in graduate school, despite this pluralism being at odds with recent administrative and professional developments we consider medicalized.

The history of how medicalization came to be an influence on counselling is multifaceted and owes something to a convergence of professionalization with scientific, political, and economic factors (Bondi

This chapter was co-authored with Konstantinos Chondros and Vanessa Vegter.

T. Strong, *Medicalizing Counselling*, Palgrave Studies in the Theory and History of Psychology, DOI 10.1007/978-3-319-56699-3_7

2004; Mendelberg 2014). The short version of that history is that many counsellors contribute to a mental *health* sector of the economy that has particular expectations on how practice is to be managed (Pearce 2014; Pilecki et al. 2011). Becoming mental health professionals enabled counsellors to be paid, regulated, and administered in ways consistent with other health-care professionals (Bergman 2013; Conti et al. 2004).

The disorders in DSMIII to today's DSM-5 became researchable in ways that diseases and injuries (and their treatment) had been in medicine, and counselling psychologists (e.g. Chwalisz 2003) advocated for a commitment to evidence-based interventions. To honor this kind of advocacy required an alignment of epistemologies between the science and the intervention approaches researched (Busch 2012). Standardization of the concerns and interventions of counselling was seemingly possible (Timmermans and Berg 2003), a standardization of practice that could also be technologized to serve administrative and regulatory requirements.

By the late 1980s, mental health software enabled clients' diagnosed conditions to be algorithmically linked to "doses" of evidence-supported interventions—an administrative godsend for making mental health practices and costs "accountable and countable" (Burton and van den Broek 2009; Sharfstein 1987a, b). These administrative algorithms align treatment for validly diagnosed disorders with treatment integrity (i.e. according to the manuals used in clinically controlled studies; see Lilienfeld et al. 2013; Park et al. 2015). Administratively, these considerations seem reasonable: a rational system of scientifically established and cost-containable care addresses what might otherwise seem like well-intended service anarchy.

Many counsellors reluctantly accept this systematized view of practice, raising ethical concerns and even going so far as to deceive administrators and funders to ensure clients get services they perceive are needed (Cooper and Gottlieb 2000; Cosgrove 2005) or to practice from preferred, non-medicalized, approaches (Strong et al. 2012; Miller 2004). While administrators and funders of counselling ration services in ways described here as medicalized (e.g. Csiernik and Csiernik 2012; Merrick et al. 2006), prospective clients also assert that "mental health" services are a priority (Evans-Lacko et al. 2012). Counsellors have railed against an audit-mindedness or loss of professional autonomy (Hage 2003; House 1996). Regardless of how such economics of mental health translate to counsellors' expected practices (Goodheart 2010), the concerns amplify with developments associated with professionally regulating counsellor practice (McGivern and Fischer 2012).

Increasingly, to be paid or managed, counsellors must address diagnosable client concerns using evidence-based treatments (Miller 2004; Zhang et al. 2013). Accordingly, to be recognized as medical or mental health professionals, counsellors have had to lobby for new forms of professional status (e.g. Bergman 2013) or rename their associations as did the CCPA (de Cicco, n.d.; from the CCA). With such a shift in professional alignment came new marketplace discourses of efficiency and accountability (Procter 2015) underpinned by an evidence-based science imported from medicine (Chwalisz 2003). Counsellors have adopted this aspect of medical practice, which some claim has become the administrative and regulatory framework under which they practice (e.g. Lees et al. 2014). For this chapter we will draw from findings of a funded (University of Calgary and Social Sciences and Humanities Research Council of Canada) study wherein we examined such medicalizing trends as they related to administering and regulating counselling, using the mapping procedures of SA (Clarke 2005; Clarke et al. 2015) to represent tensions we found in the literature, document, and website reviews, and from surveys and interviews with students and recent graduates, counsellor educators, and counselling profession leaders. We link our findings to medicalizing influences on counselling, and study details are available from the authors.

Situating Our Situational Analysis

SA was developed by Clarke (2005) as a "postmodern" response to complexities that other forms of grounded theory problematically and thematically reduced to commonalities. Missing, for Clarke, were a politics of meaning at stake in cultural developments, like those regarding the "morning after" pill's reception in America. In other words, for situations like the morning after pill's reception, she found no common themes and processes, only different social worlds, arenas, and discourse positions that became evident in studying such contested developments. We see medicalization as one such development within counselling; and its tensions and nuances warrant an examination that aims to emphasize "partialities, positionalities, complications, tenuousness, instabilities, irregularities, contradictions, heterogeneities, situatedness, and fragmentation—complexities" (Clarke 2005: xxiv). SA is a useful method for mapping human, non-human, and discursive elements involved in complex and politicized situations such as medicalizing developments in counselling. Using SA mapping techniques helped us consider and visually depict macro- and micro-level elements and influences pertaining to medicalized counselling, through identifying stakeholders invested in the situation, stakeholder discourses, and tensions related to differences over these discourses.

The first macro-look at our situation involves the mapping the groups of individuals who influence and are influenced by medicalized counselling through collective action. The visual depiction of these stakeholders is referred to in SA as a social worlds/arenas map. *Social worlds* refer to the various overlapping formal and informal collectives that organize social life (Clarke 2014). An *arena* is where the interests of multiple social worlds intersect, though these interests are often conflicting or contradicting as different discourses inform what these collectives want to accomplish (Clarke 2014). To construct our social worlds/arenas map, we conducted a review of Canadian counselling and counsellor education literature, as well as program websites, textbooks, and other curricula information related to counsellor education in Canada. While variations on the social worlds/arenas map of our situation are possible and encouraged, the intent of SA maps is not representational accuracy, generalizability, or to portray an exhaustive account. Instead, the interpretive possibilities portrayed by SA mapping enables new forms of analysis, resists concretizing simplifications, and acts as a catalyst for new forms of theorizing and dialogue (Clarke 2005). Thus, our social worlds/arenas map is a visual resource for reflecting upon who is involved in medicalized influences in counselling (see Fig. 7.1).

While this map is not exhaustive, our aim is to demonstrate the various collectives who have a stake in how counselling is conducted, and

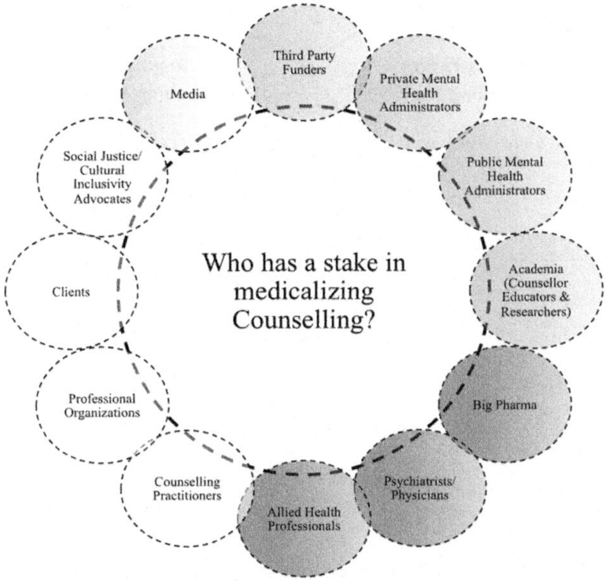
Who has a stake in medicalizing Counselling?
Third Party Funders
Private Mental Health Administrators
Public Mental Health Administrators
Academia (Counsellor Educators & Researchers)
Big Pharma
Psychiatrists/ Physicians
Allied Health Professionals
Counselling Practitioners
Professional Organizations
Clients
Social Justice/ Cultural Inclusivity Advocates
Media

Fig. 7.1 Map of social worlds in medicalizing the counselling arena

how these collectives influence and are influenced by one another and the broader situation. The dotted lines encircling these collectives (or social worlds) help to portray the overlapping, changing, and porous nature of such collectives (i.e. individuals may be members of multiple social worlds simultaneously and membership may vary over time). While the social worlds are depicted as equal in size, these worlds do not have equal influence or power. For instance, although clients are implicated and have a stake in the situation, they exert little power in influencing how counselling is conducted. Such *implicated actors*, however, may increase their power in the situation (to influence practice or other social worlds) by collectivizing, such as through forming advocacy groups. The shading of the circles is meant to represent social worlds where medicalizing discourse is presumed to be more common or expected. While we claim no quantitative basis for this shading, our decision to do so came from a review of our various data sources, including comments by our participants. This map is a visual aid for

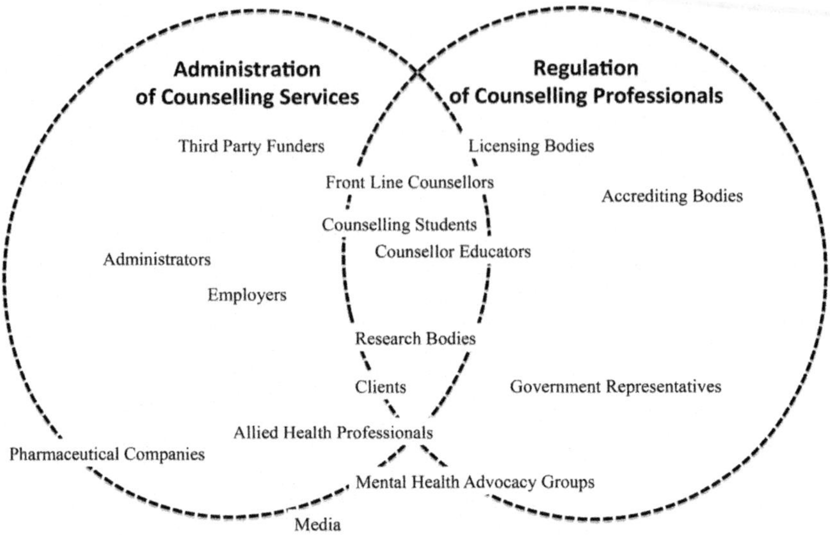

Fig. 7.2 Social worlds/arenas map of administration and regulation of counselling

considering power relations possibly relevant to medicalized counselling. As our interest in this chapter is medicalizing trends as they relate to (public and private mental health) administrators and professional organizations (that act as regulators) of the counselling profession, we zoom into our social worlds/arenas map to take a closer look at these areas (see Fig. 7.2).

Figure 7.1 helped us "zoom out" to show how the administration and regulation arenas of counselling overlap, in ways that informed further data collection. We wanted to "zoom in" further (see Fig. 7.2) and closely examine power relations and interactions between stakeholders over counselling's administration and regulation.

Medicalized Tensions in the Administration and Regulation of Counselling

Our review of medicalizing influences of administration and regulation on counselling involved an iterative process of reviewing participant survey and interview responses (counsellor educators, students of counselling, profession leaders—details on the actual study procedures are published elsewhere and available on request) and relevant literature. We identified sites of tension as "navigable," "negotiable," or "hot button" tensions. Navigable tensions were those posing medicalizing challenges participants encountered or anticipated, but were considered unproblematic. For instance, a counsellor (or counselling student) may experience tensions with peers over discourses used to justify (or not) medicalized approaches, the differences were negligible. Negotiable tensions could be talked through, but were often more fraught, such as differences with a supervisor regarding a need to adhere to medicalized requirements of practice (use of a diagnosis or EBPs). What makes such tensions fraught are perceived consequences (e.g. irreconcilable incompatibilities over preferred/desired approach, loss of professional autonomy, or a ruptured supervisory relationship). Finally, hot button tensions were those experienced as "dilemmatic." "Hot button" sites of tension were those concerned with medicalizing developments associated with the administration and/or regulation of counselling. Thus, these sites of tension merited closer examination.

"Hot button" sites of medicalized tension were identified from responses of students and recent graduates of counsellor education programs, and were associated with *professional/ethical responsibility*, *employability/registration*, and *site requirements*. We also turned to counselling profession leaders (textbook authors, members of professional organizations, long-time counselling professionals, and counsellor educators) who also identified what we analyze as hot button tensions: *administrative pressure*, *referral/accountability to allied health*, and *scope of practice/professional identity*.

By this analysis, we are not suggesting that all counsellors, profession leaders, or students will experience these tensions, or relate to such tensions in the same way (i.e. a hot button tension for one participant may be considered negotiable by another). Our participants' responses oriented us to how medicalizing discourse sometimes influences counselling, and new ways to reflect upon these influences (Clarke 2005). In examining how the administration and regulation of counsellor education increasingly moves and constrains counselling practices in a medicalized direction, we focus first on the general discourses participants used to account for what seemed at stake in how medicalizing

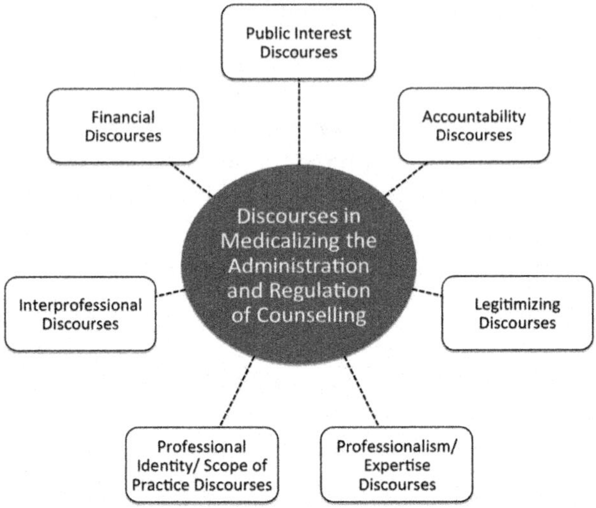

Fig. 7.3 Map of discourses in medicalizing the administration and regulation of counselling

influences the administration and regulation of counselling. These discourses highlight contested "points of view" with respect to medicalized counselling (see Fig. 7.3).

Medicalized Hot Button Tensions

While Fig. 7.3 depicts discourses relevant to counselling's administration and regulation in medicalizing ways, our hot button tensions were identified from participant comments, supplemented by analyses from the relevant professional and research literature. Employability and registration were frequently cited by students and recent graduates when trying to secure a paid position as a counsellor, or becoming a registered professional. With the shift of counselling services into the economy's mental health sector, counselling students anticipated entering a workforce wherein a medicalized approach was dominant. As one participant noted:

> It is my preference to stay away from a medicalized approach… having just been through an experience at my previous workplace in which

> funding... was tied to adherence to a medicalized approach, I have begun to accept that following a more medicalized approach may be the only way I am able to make a respectable living as a counsellor.

A "respectable" living is key here, as lower paid and more transient employment was possible with non-profit agencies not requiring medicalized approaches to practice. However, financial and professional legitimacy considerations motivated students to seek secure remuneration with public mental health organizations where they would be expected to adhere to medicalized approaches. Central to the financial tensions associated with administering these mental health services are economic concepts such as *cost-effectiveness*, *-utility*, *-benefit*, and *-offset* (Kaplan and Groessl 2002), used to justify a rationing of services in ways consistent with medicalizing discourse. Underlying both employment and administering mental health care are needs to ensure that clients can access necessary services at the lowest cost possible (Tovian 2004).

Miller (2004: 289) described tensions in counselling as stemming from administrative and regulatory pressures related to "the government's need to find accountable, credible service providers and the counselling profession's need for autonomy and professionalisation." Overlaps between administration and regulation become evident in the fact counsellors are granted access to third-party funding only if they are members of a regulated profession or established professional association (Miller and Furbish 2013). As one participant in our study noted: "We're now being kind of held accountable to the government, and we need to prove to them that we're doing best treatment practices and that we're assessing and diagnosing the clients and evaluating their addictions appropriately." The same participant went on to describe:

> a push towards getting more integrated into the mental health community and being able to have those issues appropriately addressed or assessed and diagnosed and treated... all with the sense of improving efficiency and improving treatment outcomes and all this kind of stuff. So it was through... this formal accreditation process.

A "marriage" of sorts involving the administration and regulation of counselling may have been one of convenience. To be regarded as a health profession—to confer professional legitimacy on counselling—regulatory changes were required: a code of ethics, establishing and implementing complaints/disciplinary procedures, offering continuing education credits/professional development training, and overseeing supervision processes (to do "quality control"; Miller 2004). Medicalizing discourses using DSM diagnoses and the psychological science behind EBPs provided a scientific means for how mental health could be rationally administered, legitimizing the provision of professional services to the public (Castelnuovo et al. 2016). Had psychology ignored these economic pressures governing health-care costs, the profession might have developed a dubious public reputation, jeopardizing further funding that targeted for further research, teaching, and the training of future practitioners (Goodheart 2010). Counsellors have typically not lagged behind their "elder siblings" in the field of psychology in legitimizing their professional practices.

This legitimacy relates to professional and ethical responsibility—another hot button tension with respect to counsellors' expectations and responsibilities, such as using EBPs to responsibly and accountably address clients' presenting concerns. Administering counselling is often justified according to protecting and addressing clients' concerns using the most efficient and effective procedures supported by science, mental health's EBPs, or "best practices" (Castelnuovo et al. 2016; Frank et al. 2009; Sanderson 2003). While "an imperfect science," administrative requirements for EBPs privilege standardized, symptom-reduction approaches, and sideline other counselling approaches that are less standardized and thus not amenable to measurement (McGivern and Fischer 2012). As a survey respondent stated:

> When we discussed… client "rights" to best available treatment… "best available treatment" was frequently said to be subjective in that systems of counseling that lend themselves well to being empirically studied and manualized will always have a larger evidence base than something like existential psychotherapy.

A medicalized and administrative push for using EBPs can be at odds with other counselling approaches or discourses, such as a common factors discourse. Returning to the same survey respondent: "Yet, it was emphasized to us that all systems/approaches appear to be equally effective, with greatest effects interpreted to be attributable to extra-therapy factors and the therapeutic relationship." This respondent cited the common factors view (Wampold and Imel 2015), which downplays EBPs for relational and other factors' centrality to counselling.

Site (i.e. varied contexts offering counselling) requirements were another cited source of hot button tensions. Such administrative requirements of counsellors included diagnoses, expected use of EBPs, use of brief or time-limited therapies, medically oriented record-keeping practices and assessment tools, and possible medicalized technologies. While such requirements did vary, often site requirements were non-negotiable, as one student noted: "This is our approach—you have to know it, you have to apply it." Another participant commented: "Clients must 'meet our mandate'... So if they do not fit minimums within the DSM criteria, they would not receive services here." Such can be the dilemmatic aspects that come with site requirements, regardless of the counsellor's position or approach, or the client's desire/need for services.

Site requirements inform the administration of mental health services and, even if not mandated, medicalizing discourse may be the source of administrative pressure—a hot button tension identified by our counselling profession leaders. Goodheart (2010) argued for counsellors' financial literacy, to recognize how what we have described as medicalizing discourse financially influences complex systems operating within administration and regulatory controls. These systems have public and/or private funders seeking to minimize the costs of mental health-care provision, while increasing service accessibility for clients (Goodheart 2010). From an assumption that, without services, employees' mental health could be compromised, key financial stakeholders, such as provincial health authorities, rely on EBPs as a cost-saving option for their own bottom lines, to manage mental health service budgets (Goodheart 2007).

How does such administration influence the practice of counselling? Third-party funders, for example, can restrict counsellor autonomy by funding only diagnostically based, EBP-related, cost-effective practice (Miller 1998). As one counselling profession leader remarked to us: "[Administrators] of course want to pay as little as possible, so it's an advantage to them to look at people in terms of their symptoms alone." Favored by third-party funders are standardized, brief therapy approaches, such as CBT, to address client concerns while minimizing the provider's costs. One participant suggested that: "There's an increasing amount of pressure on counsellors to do what they do in a shorter amount of time, with more complex presenting issues." The science behind these brief diagnostic and EBP treatment protocols is intentionally *general*, but client and counsellor circumstances are often *particular* in ways that are not so generalizable. Counsellor education may be seeing relevant changes to counselling curricula to reflect a growing workplace and public need for brief EBPs (see Strong et al. forthcoming). According to a counsellor educator:

> Any pressure we might feel [to teach medicalized curricula] would be as part of the ongoing effort to see counsellors recognized by insurance and FEAPs as equal in value and use to psychologists and social workers. Because they... adhere to a medicalized model, we feel somewhat compelled to educate them [counselling students] about skills and knowledge in this area in order to gain equal billing opportunities.

Such changes to third-party funding for counselling may encourage counsellor educators to revamp their curricula to include approaches "that are goal oriented, purposeful, efficient in their use of time, minimally intrusive, client-centred, inexpensive and of high quality" (Miller 2004: 291), and use the DSM "as an assessment appraisal tool for counsellors" (Miller 2004: 292). While the tensions we have discussed here are primarily administrative, they are also indicative of the overlapping administration and regulation of the profession, since regulatory bodies shape counsellor education requirements. For one counsellor educator:

> I think that the [Provincial Regulatory Body], as well as the Minister for Education, are the two huge stakeholders advocating for a program move towards a more medicalized direction... that students get thorough knowledge in a medicalized approach.

Some respondents indicated that these pedagogical shifts may follow from regulatory efforts to legitimize the counselling profession, as illustrated by a participant's remark that:

[The Provincial Regulatory Body] keeps upping the bar on trying to impress the public on how much technical knowledge we have by extending curriculums, extending supervision, mandating continuing education, and other ridiculous movements ... when it's not our level of technical knowledge that really proves is the helpful ingredient at all.

For others, such regulatory pressure was considered necessary to facilitate graduates' access to employment in an already heavily administered mental health field.

Participating in the mental health sector, counsellors join a broader network comprised of "allied health professionals"—further medicalizing the administration of counselling services. Referral/accountability to allied health professionals was identified as another hot button site of tension by counselling profession leaders; that is, challenges that arise when collaborating with and being accountable to medical and other allied health professionals. The challenge in this accountability is described by one participant who stated:

In this increased medicalization of... our profession, in this landscape... I think referring professionals, many of them subscribe to the dominant discourse... Mental health discourse, as I understand it, is thoroughly resonant with psychiatry, that's its disciplinary underpinning. So when professionals are referring different people to us [counsellors], they are often doing so with the expectation that we are on board with the, you know, the dominant discourse of the field.

The participant continued: "So it can be... a tension for counsellors, who feel some reticence or some reluctance with that ... discourse ... Will they meet the expectations of the referring professional?" Beyond funding concerns, accountability within mental health settings to medical and allied health professionals also prompts medicalizing shifts to counselling curricula, as one educator explained:

It's not because we're strong believers in the DSM, but it seems to be the common language that they [students] need to have in order to be taken seriously out in the workplace, because they're often working on

> multidisciplinary teams where… other members of the team are using that language.

Becoming mental health professionals can help ensure counsellors get paid, and that clients get services, but this comes with addressing the needs of administrative and regulatory systems (Bergman 2013; Conti et al. 2004). The medicalizing discourses of these systems constrain counsellors' abilities to practice according to their professional identity or by alternative approaches inconsistent with medicalizing discourse. In the words of one counselling profession leader regarding professional regulation within mental health services:

> Makes us fit into a particular paradigm that is diagnosis and treatment, and it is oriented with different traditions than many educational counsellors or career counsellors or guidance counsellors. There's lots of other traditions that we [counsellors] have that don't easily fit into that medical paradigm.

Such constraints on *who* counsellors are and *what* they do point to another hot button tension identified from the responses of counselling profession leaders: scope of practice and professional identity. Counselling has been a historically pluralistic profession hosting multiple theoretical orientations and models of practice. Despite pressure to adhere to medicalized approaches as mental health practitioners, participants readily distinguished between counsellors and other mental health professionals. For instance, one participant stated:

> I don't understand why counselling psychologists and counselling psychology professionals are being expected to diagnose, when it's not something that we do. It's not part of our history, it's not… it's not necessarily a fit with the people that we're serving.

Another participant suggested, "It just doesn't make sense from a counselling framework, knowing where counselling comes from, to diagnose everything. It's not what we're for." Other participants turned to alternative discourses to describe counselling clients and how they saw their approaches as incompatible with mental health's medicalized discourse.

For example, one participant saw counselling as addressing "everyday problems" as opposed to illness or disorder, stating that: "Counselling psychology looks at people and says 'These are people with problems.'" A clinical psychologist in our study took a more medical view suggesting, "This person is sick and we need to treat them to make them well." Such differences in discourses, we suggest, are tied to distinct logics and practices that shape how counselling is conducted.

Beyond expectations one uses diagnostic language as an administrative requirement, counsellors are often required to use CBT, a preferred treatment of third-party mental health service funders (Gaudiano 2008), given its cost-effective brevity. Counsellors often must explain why counselling services are warranted (a potential ethical concern if they are required to breach confidentiality), and to ensure use of economically and scientifically justifiable practices (Csiernik and Csiernik 2012; Henneberger 1994). Tensions can therefore arise when insurers and counsellors interact from discourses that may be at odds over service provision and its associated costs. Third-party funders or insurers can, for example, insist on the use of standardized measures to objectively diagnose clients' concerns, diagnoses which can be algorithmically linked to time-limited (cost-effective) EBPs (e.g. Steinwachs 1997). Such administrative frameworks for client data gathering and analysis regarding therapeutic practice facilitate expectations for financially and professionally accountable, transparent mental health service provision (Kilbourne et al. 2010). Another administrative development has been outcome-focused practice such as that adopted at the International Center for Clinical Excellence, who have developed the OpenFIT Software. As stated on the Center's website, OpenFIT "is designed for accountable care," "to integrate seamlessly with Electronic Healthcare Record systems or Case Management system," and to "Easy qualification for value based reimbursement" (https://www.centerforclinicalexcellence.com/fit-software-tools-3). Such mental health service administrative software focuses on counsellor outcomes.

It is not just insurers (i.e. typically not counsellors), however, who oversee administrative decisions; expert consultants (typically psychologists or psychiatrists) also determine or undertake quality assurance supervision specific to services counsellors are expected to provide

(Greer and Rennie 2006). While counsellors often recommend specific approaches or interventions (most commonly, CBT), these recommendations may arise because these are the approaches that get funded or are expected (see Moses 2000 or Strong et al. 2012 for analyses of such "lip service").

Managed care is an intricate system for coordinating and administering health care, while also managing and dispersing health benefits (Cooper and Gottlieb 2000). Here again, cost control must also translate to necessary and reasonable services for clients, despite minimizing costs for the managed care company (Cantor and Fuentes 2008). Sanchez and Turner (2003) highlight how managed care companies offset costs: conducting utilization reviews (reviewing services to clients to determine if continuing treatment is warranted); practicing profiling (monitoring counsellors' cost-effectiveness); implementing session limits; patient risk sharing (e.g. client copayments); "gatekeeping" (a primary care physician must authorize referral to a mental health counsellor); and using less trained and costly providers where possible. Arguments supporting managed care have both a logical sense and strong moral underpinnings: managed care promises to deliver positive outcomes, reduce inappropriate client care, decrease fraudulent and abusive practices by mental health practitioners, and manage resources responsibly (Boyle and Callahan 1995; Broskowski 1994). A perceived upside of managed care is its increased focus on prevention, on developing a continuum of mental health services, and integrating mental health within the general health-care delivery system (by fostering collaboration with primary care providers; Robinson et al. 2004). For Csiernik and Darnell (2010), however, managed care presents clinical and ethical implications. Counsellors are often prevented from providing adequate services to clients, often being denied the opportunity to offer extra sessions by clinical directors (who are less experienced in counselling), despite the fact their rates of compensation are low. For Csiernik and Darnell (2010), mental health service providers received little training or support other than on how to complete administrative forms. Cantor and Fuentes (2008: 640) echoed concerns about inadequate service:

> [M]anaged care has not been good for the business of psychology or the scope of psychological practice, and psychologists and many patients have suffered. When a managed-care company is involved in the treatment, there is a third party present in the room who expects reports on the progress of treatment and how at times even claims to have the right to review patient files.

Cantor and Fuentes (2008) expressed related concerns about adverse consequences such "care" has for establishing a therapeutic alliance. Csiernik and Csiernik (2012) asserted that having capped Employee Assistance Program (EAP) services could also be deemed unethical practice, when cost-saving is paramount:

> There is no empirical literature documenting the abuse of uncapped EAP services by counselors or employees, and this study found that in fact the average use by employees where there is no cap is lower than the average maximum caps in place. (Csiernik and Csiernik 2012: 107)

The kind of service rationing we have been describing follows from the practice of basing "cost-effective" administrative decisions on diagnoses and EBPs for treating disorders. "Disease model" rationing has been questioned for some time (Mol 2008; Wade and Halligan 2004), and it has been a logic based on trends in the global marketplace. Such administrative economies are common in our *neoliberal* era. Esposito and Perez (2014: 416) defined neoliberalism as:

> a type of order and vision of the world in which all aspects of social, cultural, and economic life are shaped by what is sometime referred to as "market rationality" – that is, evaluating the merit of all actions according to what is deemed as valuable, acceptable, or desirable by "the market."

By such a neoliberal logic, the market—in this case, for privately funded counselling services—unsurprisingly seeks cost-effective solutions, often turning to psychopharmacological treatments and proven brief strategies to restore wellness and normalcy (Filar 2014). Concerns related to people living a wholesome, fulfilling life are a *personal* responsibility; any pathologize-able concern is a *personal* concern (Ramon 2008). Mental health services have often become a business based on a profit motive. Thus, clients' concerns are addressed as "conditions largely divorced from social, economic, and political contingencies and turned into personal pathologies that can be diagnosed and treated through the allegedly value-free traditions and naturalistic methods of science and medicine" (Esposito and Perez 2014: 415). Ferraro (2016) described neoliberalism as inherent to the psy-disciplines central to providing mental health services. CBT and its "scientific" purview has been cited as one means through which counsellors might serve such a neoliberal, administrative agenda (Cabanas 2016; Rogers-Vaughan 2016).

Rationing Counselling?

Greer and Rennie (2006: 74) rhetorically wondered: what if counselling is "not simply governed by the needs and policies of payers"? What if "it plays a contributory role"? The "contributory role" pondered is difficult to quantify, though counselling of all kinds makes effective differences in clients' lives, regardless (Seligman 1995). Counselling, as we have been describing it, acquired some of its current medicalizing tensions from a convergence of science, and administrative and regulatory practices. This convergence found a further confluence with neoliberal market developments that left more than a few counsellors wondering about the service-rationing effects all of these developments had on their ways of practice (Cushman and Gilford 2000). It is too early to assess what these developments mean for counsellor education despite advocacy for EBP among counselling psychologists (Chwalisz 2003).

Counsellors, of course, need to get paid and to practice in the ways they sign on for. As mental health service providers, this might come with a cost to their pluralistic traditions of practice, despite ongoing evidence that the client outcomes are best achieved in a quality counselling relationship premised on "common factors" (Wampold and Imel 2015). What we have aimed to do with this chapter is bring together responses from the literature, counsellors, students and educators of counselling, and counselling profession leaders. These responses have focused on the influence that administrative and regulatory developments have for counsellors and their work with clients. In Chap. 8 we will turn to how medicalizing developments bring tensions to the conversational work by which counsellors engage clients. In particular, the focus will be on how such tensions are experienced, and reconciled, or not.

References

Bergman, D. M. (2013). The role of government and lobbying in the creation of a health profession: The legal foundations of counseling. *Journal of Counseling & Development, 91*(1), 61–67.

Bondi, L. (2004). 'A double-edged sword'? The professionalisation of counselling in the United Kingdom. *Health & Place, 10*(4), 319–328.

Boyle, P. J., & Callahan, D. (1995). Managed care in mental health: The ethical issues. *Health Affairs, 14*(3), 7–22.

Broskowski, A. (1994). Current mental health care environments: Why managed care is necessary. In R. L. Lowman & R. J. Resnick (Eds.), *The mental health professional's guide to managed care* (pp. 1–18). Washington: American Psychological Association.

Burton, J., & van den Broek, D. (2009). Accountable and countable: Information management systems and the bureaucratization of social work. *British Journal of Social Work, 39*(7), 1326–1342.

Busch, R. (2012). Problematizing social context in evidence-based therapy evaluation practice/governance. In A. Lock & T. Strong (Eds.), *Discursive perspectives in therapeutic practices* (pp. 245–268). Oxford: Oxford University Press.

Cabanas, E. (2016). Rekindling individualism, consuming emotions: Constructing 'psytizens' in the age of happiness. *Culture & Psychology, 22*(3), 467–480.

Cantor, D. W., & Fuentes, M. A. (2008). Psychology's response to managed care. *Professional Psychology: Research and Practice, 39*(6), 638–645.

Castelnuovo, G., Pietrabissa, G., Cattivelli, R., Manzoni, G. M., & Molinari, E. (2016). Not only clinical efficacy in psychological treatments: Clinical psychology must promote cost-benefit, cost-effectiveness, and cost-utility analysis. *Frontiers in Psychology, 7*, 563.

Chwalisz, K. (2003). Evidence-based practice: A framework for twenty-first century scientist-practitioner training. *The Counseling Psychologist, 31*(5), 497–528.

Clarke, A. E. (2005). *Situational analysis: Grounded theory after the postmodern turn*. Thousand Oaks, CA: Sage.

Clarke, A. E., Friese, C., & Washburn, R. (Eds.). (2015). *Situational analysis in practice: Mapping research with grounded theory*. Walnut Creek, CA: Left Coast Press.

Conti, R., Frank, R. G. & McGuire, T. G. (2004). Insuring mental health care in the age of managed care, In B. Lubotsky Levin, J. Petrila, & K. D. Hennessy (Eds.), *Mental health services: A public health perspective* (pp. 15–41). New York: Oxford University Press.

Cooper, C. C., & Gottlieb, M. C. (2000). Ethical issues with managed care: Challenges facing counseling psychology. *The Counseling Psychologist, 28*(2), 179–236.

Cosgrove, L. (2005). When labels mask oppression: Implications for teaching psychiatric taxonomy to mental health counselors. *Journal of Mental Health Counseling, 27*(4), 283–296.

Csiernik, R., & Csiernik, A. (2012). Canadian employee assistance programming: An overview. *Journal of Workplace Behavioral Health, 27*(2), 100–116.

Csiernik, R., & Darnell, K. (2010). Perceptions of affiliate EAP counselors: An exploratory study. *Journal of Workplace Behavioral Health, 25*(2), 154–168.

Cushman, P., & Gilford, P. (2000). Will managed care change our way of being? *American Psychologist, 55*(9), 985–996.

Esposito, L., & Perez, F. M. (2014). Neoliberalism and the commodification of mental health. *Humanity & Society, 38*(4), 414–442.

Evans-Lacko, S. E., Baum, N., Danis, M., Biddle, A., & Goold, S. (2012). Laypersons' choices and deliberations for mental health coverage. *Administration and Policy in Mental Health and Mental Health Services Research, 39*(3), 158–169.

Ferraro, D. (2016). Psychology in the age of austerity: Psychology and austerity. *Psychotherapy and Politics International, 14*(1), 17–24.

Filar, R. (2014, April 1). Mental health: Why we're all sick under neoliberalism. *Transformation*. Accessed December 29, 2016, from https://www.opendemocracy.net/transformation/ray-filar/mental-health-why-were-all-sick-under-neoliberalism.

Frank, R. G., Goldman, H. H., & McGuire, T. G. (2009). Trends in mental health cost growth: An expanded role for management? *Health Affairs, 28*(3), 649.

Gaudiano, B. A. (2008). Cognitive-behavioural therapies: Achievements and challenges. *Evidence-Based Mental Health, 11*(1), 5–7.

Gazzola, N., Smith, J. D., King-Andrews, H. L., & Kearney, M. K. (2010). Professional characteristics of Canadian counsellors: Results of a national Survey/L'identité professionnelle des conseillers canadiens: Résultats d'une enquête nationale. *Canadian Journal of Counselling, 44*(2), 83. Online.

Goodheart, C. D. (2007). Economic advocacy: What's in your wallet? *The Independent Practitioner, 27,* 129–131.

Goodheart, C. D. (2010). Economics and psychology practice: What we need to know and why. *Professional Psychology: Research and Practice, 41*(3), 189–195.

Greer, L., & Rennie, D. L. (2006). Providers' and payers' endorsements of empirically supported therapy: A power-knowledge relationship? *Psychotherapy Research, 16*(1), 67–79.

Hage, S. M. (2003). Reaffirming the unique identity of counseling psychology: Opting for the 'road less traveled by'. *The Counseling Psychologist, 31*(5), 555–563.

Henneberger, M. (1994, October 9). Managed care changing practice of psychotherapy. *New York Times*. Accessed December 29, 2016, from http://www.nytimes.com/1994/10/09/nyregion/managed-care-changing-practice-of-psychotherapy.html?pagewanted=all.

House, R. (1996). 'Audit-mindedness' in counselling. *British Journal of Guidance and Counselling, 24,* 277–283.

Kaplan, R. M., & Groessl, E. J. (2002). Applications of cost-effectiveness methodologies in behavioral medicine. *Journal of Consulting and Clinical Psychology, 70*(3), 482–493.

Kilbourne, A. M., Keyser, D., & Pincus, H. A. (2010). Challenges and opportunities in measuring the quality of mental health care. *Canadian Journal of Psychiatry, 55*(9), 549–557.

Lees, J., Macaskie, J., & Freshwater, D. (2014). Social and political perspectives on the psychotherapy and counselling profession: Returning caravelles. *European Journal of Psychotherapy & Counselling, 16*(4), 298–314.

Lilienfeld, S. O., Ritschel, L. A., Lynn, S. J., Cautin, R. L., & Latzman, R. D. (2013). Why many clinical psychologists are resistant to evidence-based practice: Root causes and constructive remedies. *Clinical Psychology Review, 33*(7), 883–900.

McGivern, G., & Fischer, M. D. (2012). Reactivity and reactions to regulatory transparency in medicine, psychotherapy and counselling. *Social Science and Medicine, 74*(3), 289–296.

Mendelberg, H. E. (2014). The integration of professional values and market demands: A practice model. *The Psychologist-Manager Journal, 17*(3), 159–177.

Merrick, E. L., Horgan, C. M., Garnick, D. W., & Hodgkin, D. (2006). Managed care organizations' use of treatment management strategies for outpatient mental health care. *Administration and Policy in Mental Health and Mental Health Services Research, 33*(1), 104–114.

Miller, J. H. (2004). Third-party funding and counselling in New Zealand: Implications for counselling services and professional autonomy. *International Journal for the Advancement of Counselling, 26*(3), 285–299.

Miller, J. H., & Furbish, D. S. (2013). Counseling in New Zealand. In T. H. Hohenshil, N. E. Amundson, & S. G. Niles (Eds.), *Counseling around the world: An international handbook*. American Counseling Association: Alexandria, VA.

Mol, A. (2008). *The logic of care: Health and the problem of patient choice*. London: Routledge.

Moses, I. (2000). Is it ethical to deceive managed care companies? A panel of the new editors of the journal of contemporary psychotherapy. *Journal of Contemporary Psychotherapy, 30*(3), 217–237.

Park, A. L., Chorpita, B. F., Regan, J., Weisz, J. R. & The Research Network on Youth Mental Health. (2015). Integrity of evidence-based practice: Are providers modifying practice content or practice sequencing? *Administration and Policy in Mental Health and Mental Health Services Research, 42*(2), 186–196.

Pearce, P. (2014). Forty years on from Rogers' APA address 'some new challenges for the helping professions. *Self & Society, 41*(2), 38.

Pilecki, B. C., Clegg, J. W., & McKay, D. (2011). The influence of corporate and political interests on models of illness in the evolution of the DSM. *European Psychiatry, 26*(3), 194–200.

Procter, G. (2015). The NHS in 2015. *Therapy Today*, 26(9): 18–25. Accessed March 1, 2016, from http://therapytoday.net/article/show/5051/the-nhs-in-2015/.

Ramon, S. (2008). Neoliberalism and its implications for mental health in the UK. *International Journal of Law and Psychiatry, 31*(2), 116–125.

Robinson, J. H., Haaz, E. J., Petrica, S. C., Hillsberg, B. S., & Kennedy, N. J. (2004). Managed care and prevention of mental health and substance abuse problems: Opportunities for growth through collaboration in the new millennium. *Journal of Primary Prevention, 24*(3), 355–373.

Rogers-Vaughn, B. (2016). *Caring for souls in a neoliberal age*. New York: Palgrave Macmillan.

Sanchez, L. M., & Turner, S. M. (2003). Practicing psychology in the era of managed care: Implications for practice and training. *American Psychologist, 58*(2), 116–129.

Sanderson, W. C. (2003). Why empirically supported psychological treatments are important. *Behavior Modification, 27*(3), 290–299.
Seligman, M. (1995). The effectiveness of psychotherapy. *The Consumer Reports Study, 50*(12), 965–974.
Sharfstein, S. S. (1987a). Reimbursement resistance to treatment and support for the long-term mental patient. *New Directions for Mental Health Services, 33,* 75–85.
Sharfstein, S. S. (1987b). Third-party payments, cost containment, and DSM-III. In G. L. Tischler (Ed.), *Diagnosis and classification in psychiatry: A critical appraisal of DSM-III* (pp. 530–538). New York: Cambridge University Press.
Steinwachs, D. M. (1997). Consumer outcomes and managed behavioral health care: Research priorities. In M. Edmunds, R. Frank, M. Hogan, D. McCarty, R. Robinson-Beale, & C. Weisner (Eds.), *Managed care: Quality improvement in behavioral health* (pp. 312–335). Washington: National Academy Press.
Strong, T., Chondros, K., Vegter, V., & Job, C. (forthcoming). Medicalizing tensions in counsellor education? *European Journal of Psychotherapy and Counselling.*
Strong, T., Gaete, J., Sametband, I. N., French, J., & Eeson, J. (2012). Counsellors respond to the DSM-IV-TR. *Canadian Journal of Counselling and Psychotherapy, 46*(2), 85–106.
Timmermans, S., & Berg, M. (2003). *The gold standard: The challenge of evidence-based medicine and standardization in health care.* Philadelphia: Temple University Press.
Tovian, S. M. (2004). Health services and health care economics: The health psychology marketplace. *Health Psychology, 23*(2), 138–141.
Wade, D. T., & Halligan, P. W. (2004). Do biomedical models of illness make for good healthcare systems? *British Medical Journal, 329*(7479), 1398–1401.
Wampold, B. E., & Imel, Z. E. (2015). *The great psychotherapy debate: The evidence for what makes psychotherapy work.* New York: Routledge.
Zhang, M., Shubina, M., Morrison, F., & Turchin, A. (2013). Following the money: Copy-paste of lifestyle counseling documentation and provider billing. *BMC Health Services Research, 13*(1), 377.

8

Tensions for Front-Line Counsellors?

What does language want of me?
(Jean-Francois Lyotard, in Lyotard and Thébaud 1996: 98)

Many readers will know Lyotard, whom I have quoted, as the author of the infamous *The Postmodern Condition: A Report on Knowledge* (Lyotard 1984). He brought the later linguistic views of Wittgenstein (1953) to this study of knowledge commissioned by universities in the province of Quebec. While his (1984) famous conclusion was that "postmodernity" meant the "end of metanarratives," it was hardly a new philosophical position. In later books, such as *The Differend: Phrases in Dispute* (Lyotard 1988) or *Just Gaming* (Lyotard and Thébaud 1996), a collection of interviews, Lyotard turned more attentively to the implications of his postmodern conclusion, examining differences in the "language games" of truth, and the ethical implications he saw arising from such differences. For those familiar with Thomas Kuhn's (1962) notion of incommensurability between scientific paradigms, the parallels will be relevant, and relate to the "reality tunnel" notion of discourse discussed in Chap. 2. Lyotard's *The Differend* elucidates the problem, addressing what seems at stake and troublesome when there is no "metalanguage"

T. Strong, *Medicalizing Counselling*, Palgrave Studies in the Theory and History of Psychology, DOI 10.1007/978-3-319-56699-3_8

to which one can turn for ultimate understanding. The ethical and practical implications of having no metalanguage—medicalizing or otherwise—in counselling partly focuses on what this chapter aims to examine.

Behind Lyotard's postmodern conclusion is a view that many discourse theorists associate with a politics of representation (e.g. Fairclough 1989; Potter 1996), though Lyotard approached language *use* from a Wittgensteinian (1953, 1969) perspective. "Language games," in Wittgenstein's sense, refer to differences in meaning associated with particular forms of language *use* in conversational interaction. From this perspective, the many approaches or discourses used by counsellors are like "language games," each with their own meanings and expected ways of talking, with overlaps between approaches (Heaton 2014). The word "game" should not be understood pejoratively, but offers insight into the normative "rules" or grammars by which any game gets played. The Rogerian language game is, by this logic, taken up by clients and counsellors in ways different from the CBT language game, or the solution-focused one. The "language game" metaphor, for Wittgenstein and Lyotard, also extended to science, and adaptations of this metaphor can be found in Latour's (1987, 2005) approach to science as well. Wittgenstein (1953) equated the languages in language games with "forms of life." Counsellors have translational and other differences to conversationally work out given differences in counselling approaches or discourses. While discourses find their coherence in common meaning, language games can be a way to more easily understand how meanings feature in micro-routines or "rules" for using and acting language consistent with discourse. Thus, medicalizing discourse follows different understandings and rules than many other counselling discourses.

In this chapter, I will adapt the language game metaphor to include (Lyotard's 1988; Lyotard and Thébaud 1996) ethical and practical considerations, and focus on tensions in the practice of counselling associated with language games common to expected use of medicalizing discourse. Tensions in this sense refer to working with discourse differences in conversational and other forms of work associated with counselling. Across many contexts of mental health practice, medicalizing discourse presumptively operates as a kind of *meta*-discourse that enables professionals and administrators to understand, use, or refer to common meanings and practices in providing care to clients. How medicalizing discourse translates for the actual conversational work or language games of counselling shall be our primary focus, particularly for counsellors whose discourses of practice may be at odds with a medicalizing discourse focused on diagnosing and treating mental disorders. Therefore, this chapter will familiarize readers with some actual medicalizing tensions I have been describing in more abstract terms up until now.

Part of our focus in this chapter will also draw from funded (University of Calgary and Social Sciences and Humanities Research Council of Canada) studies into the experiences of counsellors, counselling students, counsellor educators, and counselling profession leaders. As with Chap. 7, Clarke's (2005) SA approach was used to map the complex and contested situation of medicalizing tensions in counselling. There is little current consensus among counsellors regarding medicalizing discourse and professional practice (e.g. Hansen 2005; Rapley et al. 2011). However, apart from general critiques, little is known about tensions between a medicalizing discourse of mental health, and the pluralistic approaches and discourses of counselling practice (Cooper and McLeod 2011). We will be ethnographically "zooming in and zooming out" (Nicolini 2013) to consider big picture and small picture tensions associated with medicalizing discourse. I will link macro- and micro-influences medicalizing discourse has on counselling practice (Gale et al. 2004), to show how situated counselling practice relates to institutional or professional notions of practice (House 2004)—and vice versa. The medical tensions described link counsellors' clinical experiences and reasoning in front-line practice back to medicalizing developments and influences.

Dialogic/Monologic Differends?

The literary theorist, Mikhail Bakhtin (e.g. 1981), made stark contrasts between monologue and dialogue. A Marxist utopian who idealized the democratic and social potentials of dialogue, he also spent most of the second half of his life in the Gulag, having been at odds with

Stalin's monologic leadership (Clark and Holquist 1984). A recurring paraphrase of Bakhtin's (1981) informs what I have been referring to as "medicalizing tensions." Specifically, Bakhtin wrote as if the words in any dialogue are never fully ours, that others have claims on their meaning and on the dialogic processes by which words acquire their meaning. In this regard, meanings and conversational process are *negotiated*, and that includes how differences between discourses, such as medicalizing and other discourses of counselling, get negotiated (or not). This is a different stance on meaning and discourse than that which is typically found in critical discourse theory where the focus tends to be on how discourses can dominate meanings and practices (e.g. Fairclough 1989, 1992)—such as those of counselling. It is a stance in keeping with Lyotard's (1984, 1988) concerns for metanarratives and differends.

My discursive presumption behind "medicalizing tensions" is that counsellors negotiate discourses with clients (and administrators, etc.), and that such negotiations encompass medicalizing and other discourses (clients' *and* counsellors') when talking, listening, wordsmithing together (Strong 2006)—even in their practical reasoning. For Bakhtin and Vygotsky synthesizer James Wertsch (1991, 1998), our inner dialogues relate to our outer dialogues. The inner reasoning informing our participation in outer dialogues begins with a responsiveness to relevant outer dialogues. In other words, we learn what is possible conversationally through our interactions with others, which in turn shapes what can be inwardly possible in the self-dialogues of our reasoning and perspective-considering. This view of how "inner" discourse occurs is rhetorical all the way down (i.e. both inner and outer; see Billig 1996, 1999); how we learn to reason inwardly, as "inner dialogue," relates to how we learn to anticipate being responded to in outer dialogues. In other words, our reasoning factors in the anticipated or imagined responses of relevant others who would have something at stake in an actual version of the dialogue's process and outcomes (see Billig 1999).

On the last point, a frequently cited concern about client participation in counselling is their relative lack of power in the counselling relationship (e.g. Guilfoyle 2005). Counsellors, by this view, don't negotiate meanings and conversational processes, they dominate clients with their preferred meanings and ways of talking. Along the same lines, counsellors could be seen as dominated by medicalizing discourse in many professional contexts. By this view, neither client nor counsellor can understand or respond from anything but a dominant discourse (see Wertsch 1991) when using language to understand concerns and how to respond to them. By contrast, for heuristic and potential clinical purposes, the dialogues of counselling will be approached as situationally negotiated processes, with meanings and outcomes that would be expected to be further negotiated in circumstances where clients and counsellors live or practice. Counselling by this ideal is a context inside which clients and counsellors can at least partly step back from the hurly-burly of everyday interactions where they must justify themselves (see Shotter 1984). In counselling, clients can mindfully reflect on discourses influencing life in the hurly-burly, and contemplate discursive resources and meanings that might be successfully be used back there.

How medicalizing and other discourses are reflected upon and negotiated in counselling (i.e. between client and counsellor) relates to their use beyond the immediacies of counselling. In moving on to the study mentioned in the introduction of this chapter, Clarke's (2005) mapping procedures will be helpful in visualizing how these bigger picture negotiations of discourse relate to who has something at stake in what transpires in and from the negotiations of discourse in counselling.

Figure 8.1 is another social worlds/arenas map reproduced from Chap. 7. The data for producing this map came from a comprehensive review of the Canadian counselling and counsellor education literature, as well as website, textbook, and curricular information pertaining to counsellor education. Mapping in SA aims to catalyze new forms of theorizing and dialogue (Clarke 2005; Clarke et al. 2015). Therefore, readers are encouraged to read the map as a visual resource, to reflect upon how medicalizing discourse influences counselling.

What Fig. 8.1 tries to show is who else might have something at stake in what the counsellor says and how they might listen. In this regard, counsellors have a kind of "answerability," to use another of Bakhtin's terms (Clark and Holquist 1984), not only to clients, who increasingly understand their concerns through mental health discourse (Strong et al. 2015), but also to their professions, managers, and funders to whom they may need to be answerable on medicalizing terms.

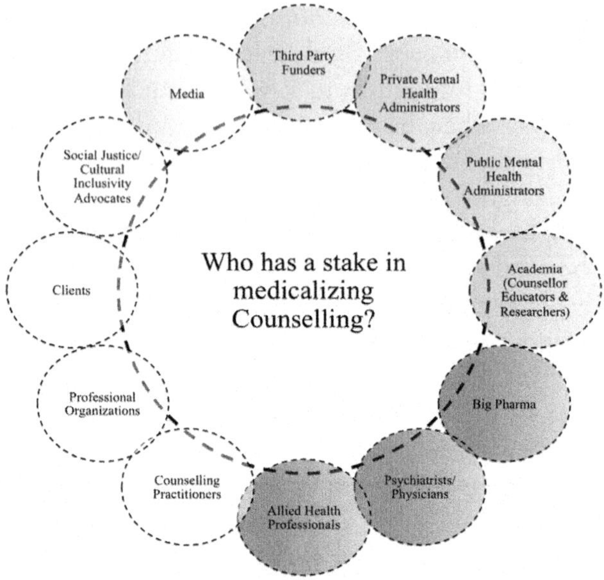
Third Party Funders
Media
Private Mental Health Administrators
Social Justice/ Cultural Inclusivity Advocates
Public Mental Health Administrators
Who has a stake in medicalizing Counselling?
Clients
Academia (Counsellor Educators & Researchers)
Professional Organizations
Big Pharma
Counselling Practitioners
Psychiatrists/ Physicians
Allied Health Professionals

Fig. 8.1 Map of social worlds in medicalizing the counselling arena

It is also important to disentangle the social worlds, from the different discourse positions circulating in situations like contemporary counselling or mental health. Discourse positions (see Harré and Slocum 2003; Harré and van Langenhove 1999) refer to being positioned within different discourses or systems of understanding and acting described in Chap. 2. Individuals, as well as social worlds and cultures, can understand and act from more than a single discourse, though it is common for discourses to dominate—with and without the awareness of those using them. The challenge is to be critically aware and resourceful—to not be used or constrained by discourse unaware, but to instead critically and resourcefully use it to intentionally position one's understanding and interacting as a counsellor. Discourse positioning theory is a resource for drawing attention to how institutions' and people's ways of responding can be constrained by either dominant or accustomed positions in discourse. This is akin to the view in narrative therapy (White and Epston 1990; Winslade 2005) that the stories people live by (i.e. are positioned within) are not the same as the people; there may be more preferred stories to live by that counselling can make accessible and negotiable in ways the client sees befitting her or his circumstances. The same can be said about discourses: that, even in the most medically oriented circumstances of counselling, different discourse positions may be accessible and negotiable. Figure 8.1 helps to highlight collectivities of actors where different discourses can be at play in the thinking and practice of counsellors and others having a stake in how counselling is practiced.

Medicalizing discourse features in the situation mapped to the extent it implicates, informs, or even dominates some of the social worlds reflected. As discussed in Chap. 7, discursive tensions arise when other discourses compete for counsellors' understandings and practices—in other words, such tensions may inform and animate counsellors', clients', and even organizations' ambivalences with respect to medicalizing discourse. From another angle, discursive tensions may also arise even if one does not use medicalizing discourse, given its often expected relevance for one's profession, work context, clients, and so on. For our analysis, it can help to see counselling as a contested conversational practice which can be variably understood and enacted. Thus, a big tension can arise should one choose to practice from pluralistic (i.e. multiple approaches) discourses over an expected single discourse of counselling (e.g. Cooper and McLeod 2012; House and Musgrave 2013). There are considerable institutional benefits to operating from a single discourse of practice, and DSM-III was seen as helping psychiatry move from using inconsistent professional and research clinical language to a more consensual (by psychiatry at least) diagnostic language (Frances 2013).

It can be useful to revisit Bakhtin's (1981) metaphor of the words (i.e. of counsellors) being not just those of counsellors. Other claims on those words can be found in the forms and records counsellors keep, but there are myriad other claims on the language or discourse counsellors use. The more obvious claims arise around such things as expected use of standardized interviews, particularly counselling approaches, diagnoses, or EBPs. In IE (Smith 2005) such expectations are tantamount to "ruling relations," or bottom lines regarding how one ought to practice—oughts that sometimes translate to counsellors practicing in unofficial ways (Strong et al. 2012). The shading of the worlds in Fig. 8.1 suggests some obvious (e.g. psychiatry) and not so obvious (e.g. media) expectations, and these can prompt reflection on when or how medicalizing tensions can influence counselling.

How these worlds converge shows how medicalizing tensions can arise over how counsellors are institutionally expected to practice and their preferred ways of practice. While it might seem clear cut that a psychiatrist would use the medicalizing discourse of DSM-5 and evidence-based interventions to diagnose and treat a client (i.e. patient), this would not preclude that psychiatrist from considering how other worlds (e.g. social justice or third-party funding) might feature in the conversational work she or he has in responding to this patient. It is the pull of these other worlds that can be the challenge on the psychiatrist's available consulting time. The psychiatrist might refer the client onto a social worker, for example, if there are concerns regarding abuse. Or, if he or she counsels from a family systems background, tensions might arise if the chosen unit to assess and work with is a couple or family (see Sutherland et al. 2016; Tomm et al. 2014). Each counselling encounter brings a convergence of such worlds, some having greater salience than others, depending on changing client, administrative context, or preferred counselling approaches. A strength-focused counsellor might work in a publicly funded mental health setting as part of an interdisciplinary team, where medication management has been central, yet rehabilitation for employment is also an expectation. What orients any consideration of the convergences of these worlds is the question of who has something at stake in how the conversations transpire; or who else has claims on the words being spoken—the assumption being that these words and ways of listening are not the counsellor's or the clients' alone, or even theirs between them.

This interchangeability of worlds and words in counselling will seem unremarkable to many counsellors. Counsellors often espouse a view of practice that suggests each counselling conversation is a cross-cultural endeavor (e.g. Monk et al. 2008; Paré 2013). The added and nuanced difference I am hoping that reference to Fig. 8.1 conveys is how these communications can have many influences and stakeholders; that a counsellor is constrained in her or his choices regarding what seems negotiable in how they listen and respond. In Chap. 2, we briefly considered metaphors of communication when discussing discourse (e.g. Turnbull 2003), and the prevailing view of communication has been a one-to-one information transmission and reception metaphor (see also Lakoff and Johnson 1980) which obscures the kinds of complexities to which I now refer. From a Bakhtinian view of counselling (see Pollard 2008), meanings that could otherwise be understood as being exchanged or shared between client and counsellor instead acquire *situational* relevance and significance. Staying with this Bakhtinian view (see also Linell 2009), while client and counsellor ostensibly talk about matters concerning the client, with counsellor responses being informed by the approach of the counsellor, a broader situation is invoked by their conversation.

It is into such situations that Fig. 8.1 offers an initial glimmer, with respect to medicalizing tensions in counselling. Clients bring with them the conversations they have been having with others, or what Harlene Anderson (1997) has referred to as "problem-organizing" conversations. To be "organized" in this sense by a problem or concern is to be affected by it in such a way that the concern focuses or dominates social interactions, and this focus of response can be from quite different standpoints (e.g. injured person, caretaker, child of injured person, neighbor, etc.). However, this is a more immediate sense of counselling than our social worlds view is getting at, where influences can be happening from a distance. Discourse theorists (e.g. Laclau and Mouffe 2001) will sometimes draw on Althusser's notion of interpellation, a term has some parallels with the Bakhtinian notion (Linell 2009) of being "answerable," in less immediate ways than face-to-face dialogue requires. The conversational work of counsellors and clients is often interpellated by expectations from the social worlds, which also have something at stake in how counselling's conversational work develops. The conversation and how it develops is not the client and counsellor's alone, obviously, particularly given that they might be answerable to a service funder's limitations, or agency practice expectations.

This is a complex view of clients and counsellors talking I have been presenting, one less focused on the immediacies of dialogue, and one inserting seeming phantom interlocutors into clients' and counsellors' conversational work together. For the hermeneutic scholar Gadamer (1988: xxviii), such complexities relate to a cultural background that shapes conversational possibilities, "over and above our wanting and doing." Figure 8.1 could be understood as a big picture and somewhat static attempt to represent fluidly relevant influences on how clients and counsellors might negotiate conversational possibilities—without seeing such influences as unidirectional (i.e. the backdrop *on* client and counsellor). Instead, what is hopefully conveyed relates to how the language used for understanding and communicating by counsellors and clients is answerable to relevant convergences of social worlds like those mapped above. A case example hopefully brings this sense out more clearly.

A client has been experiencing some despondency about his work circumstances, and has sought counselling for "stress." The counsellor, funded for an initial consultation on the client's EAP plan (Csiernik and Csiernik 2012) might have up to a further five sessions of counselling depending on her assessment of this client. Prior to seeking this consultation, the client read a colleague-recommended article on toxic workplaces, and had previously been diagnosed with an adjustment disorder with depressed mood following an ugly divorce. The counsellor in such initial consultations is expected to completed a health symptoms checklist, screen for such things as depression and medication/substance use, and decide if the client had a diagnosable condition that warranted a further five sessions of counselling, or might be more appropriately referred on to a psychiatrist. If counselling is to be offered, the counsellor must use evidence-based treatments, with progress to be evaluated by symptom checklists provided and in turn monitored by the client's EAP. The client's despondency is relatively recent and related to requirements for extra hours of work, in a "toxic" downsizing circumstance where colleagues were recently laid off. The counsellor practices from a feminist and client-centered approach focused on empowerment and meaning—an approach the EAP has cited as being insufficiently "evidence-based," even for adjustment disorders, though these disorders merit a single session and not the usual five sessions a depressed or anxious client might warrant.

Beyond the client and counsellor conversing about the client's workplace despondency, it is clear that other worlds have an influence on the words both choose, and how their conversation might progress. "Over and above" their conversation are constraints on plausible ways to make sense of the client's despondency, the official language needed for the EAP paperwork and expected EBP, and the financial relationships both client and counsellor have with their respective employers. Despite his workplace concerns, the client's reading helped him find a plausible and legitimizing (i.e. symptom-based) articulation of his despondency, as did his prior diagnosed adjustment disorder. Plausibility meant something different for the counsellor. There were her feminist and Rogerian understandings of the client's presenting concern, but also translational issues required for the EAP's medically oriented paperwork and hoped-for approval of the sessions she had planned to provide for the client. Through the Bakhtinian lens (e.g. Linell 2009; Pollard 2008), the words of both client and counsellor were not their words alone, what they could talk into significance between them was shaped to some extent by their answerability to other social worlds in which they participated. How this client and counsellor talked, and what came from their conversation, had meanings and implications in and for these other social worlds, the medicalizing one of the EAP being among the more relevant of the worlds to which they were to answer.

The complexities don't stop with such convergences of social worlds, they are also activated by different discourses that animate and inform interactions between members of different social worlds. Bring counsellors together to discuss their work, and this becomes obvious. Several decades ago, family therapist Al Scheflen (1978) described a conversation a group of counsellors had about what a client's smile meant to them, and how they would respond to that smile. A counsellor's response informed by psychodynamic discourse (or approach) would cue up a different response than another counsellor's response informed by systemic or behavioral discourse of practice. Discourses in this sense invoke ways of differently understanding and responding to developments in counselling. For Scheflen's smiling client, such discourses for understanding and responding invoke potential tensions as well. Scheflen's article was in part about "doctrinal" (i.e. discursive) differences in how these counsellors would debate such things as a client's smile. At a personal level, counsellors usually reconcile such discourse differences in counselling and in their discussions with colleagues unproblematically. Historically, most counsellors have professed eclecticism as their choice of approaches, or what I have been referring to as counselling discourses (see Cooper and McLeod 2011, 2012; Smith 1982).

Of course, such discourse differences are not restricted to counsellors; other kinds of discourse differences play out in the other, earlier mapped social worlds (consider portraying academics as all being on the same page in discourse terms, and the point is made). Professions, funders of counselling, researchers, client advocacy groups, and allied health professionals exemplify social worlds where differences occur over the discourses informing the understandings and practices of each social world. Figure 8.1, debates in the psychiatry world over diagnostic language and related science (Frances 2013; Insel 2013) interpellate further tensions within the worlds of publicly and privately funded mental health services. Responding to such differences has been a normal part of the counselling practitioner's world, though an added tension has come with what I have been describing as medicalizing discourse.

Social constructionist theorist Ken Gergen (2009) suggests discursive differences pose a challenge for people to resourcefully *coordinate* new ways to respectfully respond to each other. From an administrative standpoint, such coordinations of discourse can be costly and inconvenient. A mental health (mono)culture, based on DSM diagnoses and EBPs, purportedly legitimizes professional service under a common discourse of practice (Abbott 1988), but mental health was never comprised of a single counselling profession. Nor has there been consensus among mental health professionals regarding administratively expected uses of DSM diagnoses and EBP (e.g. Raskin and Gayle 2016).

What has been increasingly clear is that mental health concerns are now regarded as a primary health-care expense (Roehrig 2016). Despite recommendations to expand health services through the Affordable Care Act in the US (Knickman et al. 2016; Mechanic 2012), considerable cost-containment pressure has translated to more use of physician-delivered care, whether through prescribed medication use or through primary care visits (Pomerantz 2006). For counsellors, cost-containment concerns have prompted private insurers to embrace the abstract yet programmable generalizations of medicalizing discourse—in ways that reductively distort what occurs in the immediacies of counselling (e.g. APA Presidential Task Force on Evidence-Based Practice 2006; Cushman and Gilford 2000). So, while a medicalizing discourse of DSM diagnoses and evidence-based treatments helps to administer and coordinate mental health services, inflexible use of this medicalizing discourse creates tensions for counselling's conversational (Huett and Goodman 2012; Wright et al. 2012).

Discursive Positions on Medicalizing Discourse

Returning to the research that yielded Fig. 8.1, we turn now to how discourses, like medicalizing discourse, differently featured in the surveys, interviews, website and literature reviews, and other data produced from the research. While specifics of how the research was conducted can be found elsewhere (Strong et al. 2012, 2015, forthcoming-a, b), the data was obtained from counsellors, counsellor educators, students of counselling, profession leaders, graduate counsellor education curricula and websites, and literatures pertaining to counsellor training. The primary question informing the research pertained to how medicalizing discourse was experienced and responded to in counselling, and in counsellor education. The premise was that DSM diagnoses and evidence-based interventions were relatively recent to the counselling and counsellor education landscape, so curiosity focused on what this meant for a professional practice and education that historically has been pluralistic (Cooper and McLeod 2011). The aim of this qualitative research was not to produce generalizable results representative of Canadian counselling, but to offer glimpses into "medicalizing tensions." Self-selecting participants in these studies chose to be part of the research knowing they were being asked to comment on the influence of the DSM and EBP on counselling or counsellor education.

The data were analyzed using procedures from SA (Clarke 2005; Clarke et al. 2015) and this involved first identifying "elements" that were recurring and salient across the data sources. Specifically, we looked for things cited in the surveys, interviews, websites, and textbooks that spoke to the influence that medicalizing (diagnose and treat) discourse had on the learning or practice of counselling. Of particular interest were elements cited in ways that highlighted or spoke to medicalizing tensions with respect to non-medicalized discourses of counselling. Such elements included how client concerns were understood, how quality services might be provided, and counselling interventions or approaches used. Elements in our analyses were not specific to worlds and could be understood and discussed using varied discourses. For example, one can refer generally to client "concerns" (i.e. as they experienced them) and secondarily (i.e. for analytic purposes) about how discourses inform understanding or responding to such "concerns."

For the most part, the analyses undertaken for these modest studies showed that counselling continued to be learned and practiced in pluralistic ways. Graduate students across Canadian counsellor education programs, for example, tended to indicate that they learned a plurality of common counselling approaches while also learning about EBP. Similarly, counsellors described a range of practice experiences that only sometimes translated to specific tensions with a medicalizing discourse practices. Textbooks and counsellor education program websites also typically portrayed counselling in pluralistic terms. On first analysis, the kinds of medicalizing tensions described up to this point seemed insignificant.

For students, such medicalizing tensions were seldom evident until they were in assessment or practicum courses that put them out into diverse contexts of practice. For counsellor educators and profession leaders, discussion of medicalizing discourse tended to be more abstract and pertaining to general changes they associated with the then (2012–2103) incoming DSM-5. There were three primary and recurring places where data sources indicated or participants reported encountering medicalizing tensions of varied intensity: (a) in the administrative procedures and paperwork expected of them; (b) in communications with colleagues and referring professionals; and (c) in assessing how clients presented their concerns.

Where participants or sources had the most to say about medicalizing influences was with respect to administrative expectations, such as completing necessary paperwork, or in legitimizing their work as either being reimbursable or falling within agency or public service mandates. In the most medicalized of contexts, participants described feeling torn about stigmas associated with diagnosing a DSM disorder, while also recognizing that such a diagnosis enabled services that wouldn't otherwise be provided. In some cases, screening for psychopathology was a means to make referrals on for medication-oriented treatments. Some counsellors spoke of translating DSM diagnoses for concerns clients presented, in ways akin to saying "this" is how a psychiatrist would understand their concern, or that "this" would be a symptom-based way for making sense of their concern. These translational issues were not as tension-inducing as those circumstances where administrative requirements were at odds with counsellors' preferred ways of practice. This might occur when solution-focused or strengths-oriented counsellors had to assess (i.e. converse about) symptoms and skill deficits. For counsellors oriented to social justice issues, squaring their conversations with a more symptom-focused diagnostic and treatment conversation was also a source of tension. Some spoke of "playing the game" or keeping "two sets of books," which meant completing required paperwork and affixing a diagnosis, while continuing to practice in ways that did not align with medicalizing discourse—in other words, having to use diagnostic language and evidence-based interventions "officially," while using their preferred approaches unofficially. Participants also spoke of how clients' voices were sometimes usurped or subordinated by the need for their conversational work to be conducted according to administrative protocols associated with medicalizing discourse. The chief tensions related to how these administrative expectations constrained what could be "legitimately" talked about when the counsellors' approaches did not align with such medicalizing expectations.

A related tension arose in how medicalizing discourse was expected (or not) in discussions with colleagues, particularly referring professionals. Most counsellors preferred to arrive at their own formulation of the clients' concerns but this proved additionally challenging when clients came to be treated for something already diagnosed, or when their ways of formulating client concerns were at odds with a default medicalizing discourse of DSM diagnoses and evidence-based treatments. One participant spoke of needing "two faces," so she could participate in what she saw as disrespectful conversations about clients, while retaining the views of them that she would retain for her actual (somewhat covert) work with them from a non-medicalizing approach. In team-based meetings, some counsellors described finding it difficult to contest colleagues' dominant medicalizing ideas given their alternative approaches.

Sometimes the greatest challenges arose when clients presented in medicalizing discourse, and counsellors wanted to widen the conversational focus to include other discourses that might also plausibly speak to a client's concern. Narrative therapists (e.g. White 2007) have spoken of a tendency that a particular understanding, like a diagnosis or prescribed treatment, can "totalize" a client's sense of themselves and their possibilities. Counsellors often preferred to not restrict conversations to medicalizing discourse, and this could present issues in their therapeutic relationships, particularly if clients thought their medicalized understanding was being delegitimized. One participant stated, "the clients' voice is the largest voice in the room," but then wondered what that would mean with respect to how what was said by that client being translated to, or accounted for by, medicalizing discourse.

These may seem like mundane "tensions" I have been describing, and they were reported by self-selecting (for the studies) counsellors, counsellor educators, and profession leaders. For some, the tensions were more visceral or contested than for others, with some counsellors self-identifying as being professionally misaligned with workplace expectations. Some were fine with how DSM language and EBP gave both structure and scientific legitimacy to their ways of counselling, or envisioning how counselling ought to be done. In other contexts, however, participants described feeling torn over approaches to practice that formulated clients' concerns as medical in orientation, and therefore needing particular kinds of "treatment." These medicalizing tensions were most pronounced among counsellors who listened and responded to clients through meaning, strengths-focused, and systemic-relational approaches.

Reflections

> What we do is to bring words back from their metaphysical to their everyday use. (Wittgenstein 1953: 116)

Throughout this chapter, my focus has been on how the words and actions used in counselling are dialogically negotiated (Linell 2009; Pollard 2008) between clients, counsellors, and institutional and cultural influences, in the conversational work of counselling. This negotiated sense of dialogue is participatory in that we can't use words or act in any way we wish, as we are answerable to others who have claims on the words we may be using. To heighten the tensions raised with a starker contrast, a critical view of counselling is that it could be understood as a professionally directed exchange of monologues, to be practiced in ways that needn't heed the expectations of the counsellor's practice setting, professional ethics, or client preferences. I rhetorically resort to such a stark contrast, to highlight the negotiated sense of dialogue that goes with tensions as I have been describing them. Dialogue's interactional immediacies and exigencies in counselling tend to be taken for granted (Shotter 1993). Recognizing that, and how others have claims on our words and conversational processes, such conversational immediacies and exigencies (i.e. tensions) become more palpable.

The extent to which medicalizing discourse competes with other discourses (e.g. those of counselling approaches, social justice, or even spiritual discourses) for how counsellors might listen and respond to clients clearly varies by situation and client. Scientific and administrative developments associated with mental health—the primary service context where counselling services are offered—influence what is legitimate to discuss and document in counselling, as discussed in previous chapters. With funding for both publicly (Johnson 2016) and privately funded (Csiernik et al. 2016) counselling services in decline, the diagnostic and treatment algorithms associated with medicalizing discourse provide a means to ration services on the basis of symptom severity. Literally, a counsellor's pay (Moses 2000; Wylie 1995) or professionalism (Chwalisz 2003) can seem to depend on addressing such legitimacies, and this comes before what media-informed clients (Illouz 2008; Jutel 2011) also expect in their conversations with counsellors. Such tensions over what gets said and heard in counselling is a normal challenge in counselling; counsellors answer to clients—and, by extension, to fee-payers and administrators, and to counsellors' approaches or discourses of practice. Participants and data sources indicated medicalizing tensions arise over counsellor-perceived incompatibilities between a medicalizing discourse of practice and their preferences in undertaking the situated conversational work of counselling. We turn in Chap. 9 to counselling's future, to how the next generation of counsellors are being trained and supervised, and how medicalizing discourse influences that training.

References

Abbott, A. (1988). *The system of professions: An essay on the division of expert labor*. Chicago: University of Chicago Press.

Anderson, H. (1997). *Conversation, language, and possibilities: A postmodern approach to therapy*. New York: Basic Books.

APA Presidential Task Force on Evidence-Based Practice and American Psychological Association. (2006). Evidence-based practice in psychology. *American Psychologist, 61*(4), 271–285.

Bakhtin, M. (1981). *The dialogic imagination: Four essays by M.M. Bakhtin*. Austin: University of Texas Press.

Billig, M. (1996). *Arguing and thinking: A rhetorical approach to social psychology*. Cambridge: Cambridge University Press.

Billig, M. (1999). *Freudian repression: Conversation creating the unconscious*. New York: Cambridge University Press.

Chwalisz, K. (2003). Evidence-based practice: A framework for twenty-first century scientist-practitioner training. *The Counseling Psychologist, 31*(5), 497–528.

Clark, K., & Holquist, M. (1984). *Mikhail Bakhtin*. Cambridge, MA: Belknap/Harvard University Press.

Clarke, A. E. (2005). *Situational analysis: Grounded theory after the postmodern turn*. Thousand Oaks, CA: Sage.
Clarke, A. E., Friese, C., & Washburn, R. (Eds.). (2015). *Situational analysis in practice: Mapping research with grounded theory*. Walnut Creek, CA: Left Coast Press.
Cooper, M., & McLeod, J. (2011). *Pluralistic counselling and psychotherapy*. Thousand Oaks, CA: Sage.
Cooper, M., & McLeod, J. (2012). From either/or to both/and: Developing a pluralistic approach to counselling and psychotherapy. *European Journal of Psychotherapy & Counselling, 14*(1), 5–17.
Csiernik, R., & Csiernik, A. (2012). Canadian employee assistance programming: An overview. *Journal of Workplace Behavioral Health, 27*(2), 100–116.
Csiernik, R., Darnell, K., & Trotter, M. L. (2016). From the outside looking out: A qualitative examination of the experiences of Canadian external EAP providers. *EASNA Research Notes, 5*(3), 1–7.
Cushman, P., & Gilford, P. (2000). Will managed care change our way of being? *American Psychologist, 55*(9), 985–996.
Fairclough, N. (1989). *Language and power*. Harlow: Longman.
Fairclough, N. (1992). *Discourse and social change*. Cambridge: Polity Press.
Frances, A. (2013). *Saving normal: An insider's revolt against out-of-control psychiatric diagnosis, DSM-5, big pharma, and the medicalization of ordinary life*. New York: William Morrow.
Gadamer, H. G. (1988). *Truth and method* (2nd Rev. ed, J. Weinsheimer & D. G. Marshall, Trans.). London: Continuum.
Gale, J., Lawless, J., & Roulston, K. (2004). Discursive approaches to clinical research. In T. Strong & D. Paré (Eds.), *Furthering talk: Advances in the discursive therapies* (pp. 125–144). New York: Kluwer Academic/Plenum.
Gergen, K. J. (2009). *An invitation to social construction* (2nd ed.). Thousand Oaks, CA: Sage.
Guilfoyle, M. (2005). From therapeutic power to resistance? Therapy and cultural hegemony. *Theory & Psychology, 15*(1), 101–124.
Hansen, J. T. (2005). Truth or consequences: A neopragmatic critique of contemporary mental health culture. *Journal of Mental Health Counseling, 27*(3), 210–220.
Harré, R., & Slocum, N. (2003). Disputes as complex social events: On the uses of positioning theory. *Common Knowledge, 9*(1), 100–118.
Harré, R., & Van Langenhove, L. (1999). *Positioning theory: Moral contexts of intentional action*. Oxford: Blackwell.

Heaton, J. M. (2014). *Wittgenstein and psychotherapy: From paradox to wonder*. London: Palgrave Macmillan.

House, R. (2004). *Therapy beyond modernity: Deconstructing and transcending profession-centred therapy*. London: Karnac.

House, R., & Musgrave, A. (2013). 'Pluralistic accountability' for the psychological therapies? Holding the tension between diversity's virtues and the need for accountability. *British Journal of Guidance and Counselling, 41*(1), 24–35.

Huett, S. D., & Goodman, D. M. (2012). Levinas on managed care: The (a) proximal, faceless third-party and the psychotherapeutic dyad. *Journal of Theoretical and Philosophical Psychology, 32*(2), 86–102.

Illouz, E. (2008). *Saving the modern soul: Therapy, emotions, and the culture of self-help*. Berkeley: University of California Press.

Insel, T. (2013). *Post by former NIMH director Thomas Insel: Transforming diagnosis*. Accessed November 18, 2016. https://www.nimh.nih.gov/about/directors/thomas-insel/blog/2013/transforming-diagnosis.shtml.

Johnson, S. (2016, December 6). 'I left to save myself': The reality of working in children's mental health. *The Guardian*. Accessed December 13, 2016. https://www.theguardian.com/healthcare-network/2016/dec/06/reality-working-child-mental-health-services.

Jutel, A. G. (2011). *Putting a name to it: Diagnosis in contemporary society*. Baltimore: Johns Hopkins University Press.

Knickman, J., Krishnan, R., & Pincus, H. (2016). Improving access to effective care for people with mental health and substance use disorders. *JAMA, 316*(16), 1647–1648.

Kuhn, T. S. (1962). *The structure of scientific revolutions*. Chicago: University of Chicago Press.

Laclau, E., & Mouffe, C. (2001). *Hegemony and socialist strategy: Towards a radical democratic politics* (2nd ed.). New York: Verso.

Lakoff, G., & Johnson, M. (1980). *Metaphors we live by*. Chicago: University of Chicago Press.

Latour, B. (1987). *Science in action*. Cambridge, MA: Harvard University Press.

Latour, B. (2005). *Reassembling the social: An introduction to actor-network-theory*. Oxford: Oxford University Press.

Linell, P. (2009). *Rethinking language, mind, and world dialogically: Interactional and contextual theories of human sense-making*. Charlotte, NC: Information Age Publishing.

Lyotard, J. F. (1984). *The postmodern condition: A report on knowledge*. Minneapolis: University of Minnesota Press.
Lyotard, J. F. (1988). *The differend: Phrases in dispute*. Minneapolis: University of Minnesota Press.
Lyotard, J. F., & Thébaud, J. L. (1996). *Just gaming* (W. Godzich, Trans.). Minneapolis: University of Minnesota Press.
Mechanic, D. (2012). Seizing opportunities under the affordable care act for transforming the mental and behavioral health system. *Health Affairs, 31*(2), 376–382. Project Hope.
Monk, G., Winslade, J., & Sinclair, S. (2008). *New horizons in multicultural counseling*. Thousand Oaks, CA: Sage.
Moses, I. (2000). Is it ethical to deceive managed care companies? A panel of the new editors of the journal of contemporary psychotherapy. *Journal of Contemporary Psychotherapy, 30*(3), 217–237.
Nicolini, D. (2013). *Practice theory, work, and organization: An introduction*. Oxford: Oxford University Press.
Paré, D. (2013). *The practice of collaborative counseling and psychotherapy: Developing skills in culturally mindful helping*. Los Angeles: Sage.
Pollard, R. (2008). *Dialogue and desire: Mikhail Bakhtin and the linguistic turn in psychotherapy*. London: Karnac.
Pomerantz, J. M. (2006). Changing pattern of mental health service favors primary care, medication use. *Drug Benefit Trends, 18*(2), 652–653.
Potter, J. (1996). *Representing reality*. Thousand Oaks, CA: Sage.
Rapley, M., Moncrieff, J., & Dillon, J. (2011). *De-medicalizing misery: Psychiatry, psychology and the human condition*. New York: Palgrave Macmillan.
Raskin, J. D., & Gayle, M. C. (2016). DSM-5: Do psychologists really want an alternative? *Journal of Humanistic Psychology, 56*(5), 439–456.
Roehrig, C. (2016). Mental disorders top the list of the most costly conditions in the United States: $201 billion. *Health Affairs, 35*(6), 1130–1135.
Scheflen, A. E. (1978). Susan smiled: On explanation in family therapy. *Family Process, 17*(1), 59–68.
Shotter, J. (1984). *Social accountability and selfhood*. New York: Cambridge University Press.
Shotter, J. (1993). *Conversational realities*. Thousand Oaks, CA: Sage.
Smith, D. (1982). Trends in counseling and psychotherapy. *American Psychologist, 37*(7), 802–809.
Smith, D. E. (2005). *Institutional ethnography: A sociology for people*. New York: Altamira Press.

Strong, T. (2006). Wordsmithing in counselling? *European Journal of Psychotherapy and Counselling, 8*(3), 251–268.

Strong, T., Gaete, J., Sametband, I. N., French, J., & Eeson, J. (2012). Counsellors respond to the DSM-IV-TR. *Canadian Journal of Counselling and Psychotherapy, 46*(2), 85–106.

Strong, T., Ross, K. H., & Sesma-Vazquez, M. (2015). Counselling the (self?) diagnosed client: Generative and reflective conversations. *British Journal of Guidance and Counselling, 43*(5), 598–610.

Strong, T., Vegter, V., & Chondros, K. (forthcoming-a). Medicalizing tensions in counsellor education? Counselling and counselling psychology students' views. *Canadian Journal of Counselling and Psychotherapy.*

Strong, T., Chondros, K., Vegter, V., & Job, C. (forthcoming-b). Medicalizing tensions in counsellor education? *European Journal of Psychotherapy and Counselling.*

Sutherland, O., Couture, S., Gaete Silva, J., Strong, T., Lamarre, A., & Hardt, L. (2016). Social justice oriented diagnostic discussions: A discursive perspective. *Journal of Feminist Family Therapy, 28*(2–3), 76–99.

Tomm, K., St. George, S., Wulff, D., & Strong, T. (Eds.). (2014). *Patterns in interpersonal interactions: Inviting relational understandings for therapeutic change.* New York: Routledge.

Turnbull, W. (2003). *Language in action: Psychological models of conversation.* New York: Psychology Press.

Wertsch, J. V. (1991). *Voices of the mind.* Cambridge, MA: Harvard University Press.

Wertsch, J. V. (1998). *Mind as action.* Oxford: Oxford University Press.

White, M. (2007). *Maps of narrative practice.* New York: W.W. Norton.

White, M., & Epston, D. (1990). *Narrative means to therapeutic ends.* New York: W.W. Norton.

Winslade, J. M. (2005). Utilising discursive positioning in counselling. *British Journal of Guidance and Counselling, 33*(3), 351–364.

Wittgenstein, L. (1953). *Philosophical investigations* (G. E. M. Anscombe, Trans). Oxford: Basil Blackwell.

Wittgenstein, L. (1969). *On certainty.* Oxford: Blackwell Publishing.

Wright, T., Simpson-Young, V., & Lennings, C. (2012). Therapeutic process in the context of third party determined time limits. *Clinical Psychologist, 16*(2), 82–92.

Wylie, M. S. (1995). Diagnosing for dollars? *Family Therapy Networker, 19*(3), 22–23.

9

Tensions in Training Counsellors?

Teachers open the door. You enter by yourself.
Chinese Proverb

We are born into a world in conversation and learn different ways to join and extend some of these conversations. Counselling, a profession where conversation is central, has many conversational traditions or discourses of practice. As someone who teaches in a graduate counsellor education program there is always a challenge of learning to practice in professionally accepted ways. For many students this can initially translate into binary (yes/no) thinking on what counselling legitimately means. While they get exposed to the great theories or conversational traditions of counselling (e.g. Corsini and Wedding 2010), they also encounter knowledge and research methods that scientifically legitimize some counselling practices over others. In this chapter we will consider the current state and possible future of counselling and counsellor education, examining tensions within the academy for students and educators.

Universities have increasingly become the legitimizer of accepted professional wisdom and practice in counselling, or what it means to effectively engage clients in counselling's conversational work. That work

T. Strong, *Medicalizing Counselling*, Palgrave Studies in the Theory and History of Psychology, DOI 10.1007/978-3-319-56699-3_9

takes on very different meanings and practices depending on the discourses informing it, with medicalizing discourse being one of many discourses used and learned by counselling students. In this chapter 1 will confine my comments on counsellor education to learning occurring in counselling and counselling psychology Master's degree programs, recognizing that there are many other contexts in which professionals learn counselling knowledge and skills (e.g. social work, psychiatric nursing). While typically, in Canada, counselling psychologists would have doctoral-level training, Master's-level counsellor education programs often adopt curricula partly based on applying psychological knowledge. Professional definitions of practice can translate to some educational differences and related medicalizing tensions we will discuss in this chapter:

> *Canadian Counselling and Psychotherapy Association* (CCPA, n.d.): "Counselling is a relational process based upon the ethical use of specific professional competencies to facilitate human change. Counselling addresses wellness, relationships, personal growth, career development, mental health, and psychological illness or distress."
>
> *Counselling Psychology Chapter of the Canadian Psychological Association* (CPA, n.d.): "Counselling psychology is … concerned with using psychological principles to enhance and promote the positive growth, well-being, and mental health of individuals, families, groups, and the broader community."
>
> *American Counseling Association* (ACA, n.d.): "Professional counseling is a professional relationship that empowers diverse individuals, families, and groups to accomplish mental health, wellness, education, and career goals."

In this chapter, I want to present my insider's view of counsellor education, drawing from prior research (see Strong et al. 2015, 2017, forthcoming b), but also from insider debates shaping the future of counselling, on what preparation for the profession should entail. As Abbott (1988: 56–57) suggested decades ago, "the academic knowledge system of a profession generally accomplishes three tasks—legitimation, research, and instruction—and in each it shapes the vulnerability of professional jurisdiction to outside interference." Counsellor educators engage in all three profession-defining tasks, but Abbott's mention of vulnerability, in this case to requirements of a medicalizing mental health culture, will focus attention in this chapter.

Some have referred to counselling as a "gatekeeping profession" (Erickson and Shultz 1982; or for a more recent, student view, Foster, Leppma, and Hutchinson 2014), and, by extension, that would make counsellor educators potential gatekeepers of gatekeepers. While Erickson and Schultz were focused on mostly counselling within educational settings, their interest was with the face-to-face conversational work of counselling, particularly on the influence counsellors had on students' futures as they conversed. Consequential things also get discussed in the many conversations of counsellor education, extending to how counsellor educators discuss the profession's future with each other.

In the profession's early days, a primary training focus was on developing attributes and personality traits of counsellors-in-training, and on technical or relational skills (e.g. Cottle 1953; Cox 1945; Tyler 1953; Wright and Darley 1947). With Carl Rogers' seminal (1941)book, *Counseling and Psychotherapy*, counsellors took a greater relational focus in their work, while techniques and other therapeutic factors remained a scientific curiosity (Hathaway 1948). Part of this focus would change with behavioral developments that informed learning and counsellor training (see Carkhuff 1967). By the 1970s, Carl Rogers (1973) was still expressing his longstanding concerns over counselling becoming an overly technical profession too rooted in outdated philosophies and insufficiently open to a full range of human experience and potential. Counsellor education, like other forms of professional education informed by social science, has seen its share of trends and bandwagons, some narrowing counselling's scope more than others.

Relationships, Common Factors, and Competencies in Counselling?

What makes for good counselling or good counsellors has been a contested notion for decades. Different metaphors animating professional discussions in critical psychology have been part of the contest.

A "McDonaldization" of counselling based on standardizing learning and expected practices is seen by recent critics as abandoning important traditions while addressing marketplace requirements for evidence-based brief interventions (Goodman 2016). Paralleling these concerns, some educators in clinical psychology recently warned of a narrowing of practice orientations to a focus on CBT (Heatherington et al. 2012). Counselling psychologists tend not to be far behind their clinical psychology colleagues when it comes to such developments (Ogunfowora and Drapeau 2008). In training counsellors for professional practice, the social science legitimizing and informing graduate student education is central to preparing graduates for the conversations they, as future counsellors, will have with their clients.

A big debate across counselling approaches has been over how much practice and, by extension, training should focus on discrete evidence-based interventions over "common factors" (Duncan et al. 2010; Wampold et al. 2017) that are more relationally and conversationally focused (i.e. closer to where Rogers was coming from). At the start of this chapter definitions of counselling and counselling psychology differently emphasize these practice and training foci. This is despite a recurrent finding from client evaluations regarding counselling effectiveness, that the "common factors" (patient engagement, affective experiencing, and therapeutic alliance) are rated most helpful, rather than specific interventions or applications of psychological knowledge. Of course, counsellors are not alone in developing supportive relationships; paraprofessionals have been identified as helpful, calling into question whether graduate-trained counsellors offer clients anything better (Durlak 1979). Where training of graduate-level counsellors appears to make a difference is in negotiating with clients more precise tasks, such as a focus for counselling (Berman and Norton 1985; Mallinckrodt and Nelson 1991). While a research focus persists on identifying and measuring specific psychological interventions or actions taken by counsellors to enhance clients' lives (i.e. causal factors of change), common factors and other non-specific aspects remain central to the profession's definition of counselling (e.g. CPA, n.d.).

Regardless, considerable attention has focused on specific competencies counsellors are expected to develop and demonstrate (e.g. Menne

1975; Sue et al. 1992), with similar competencies now articulated for supervisors of counsellors (Neuer Colburn et al. 2016). Such a focus on competencies has facilitated the development of standardized, learnable, and measurable micro-skills that play an important role in training counselors (e.g. Ivey et al. 1993). Even dimensions of counselling referred to as "common factors" have been translated into a taxonomy of instructable and measurable competencies (Tschacher et al. 2014). Less clear, however, has been the importance of other applications of psychological knowledge to good counselling.

Guidance and Developmental Tasks?

Recall that the early decades of professional counselling were often focused on providing "guidance" (Hoyt 1962). A question can arise from this focus: on what basis should guidance be offered? The answers to this question have varied but an early line of response was that guidance and counselling should target the accomplishment of developmental milestones. The psychology of human development became helpful in identifying norms against which clients' development could be assessed, and in identifying developmental tasks to attain educational and counselling purposes (Havighurst 1948). This focus on developmental tasks, associated with normative processes and milestones, was widely taken up by counsellors to understand and facilitate vocational development (Super 1953), relationship development (Carter and McGoldrick 1980), and even bereavement (Worden 1991). This view of normative development also related to school psychology's emphasis on psychological assessment and educational remediation, dating back to the development of early intelligence measures (e.g. Binet 1916). It is a view that fits well with theoretical (Boorse 1977) as well as lay conceptions of health considered departures from normal (i.e. normative) quality-of-life experiences.

The developmental framework was useful for initially linking psychology to counselling in realizing Abbott's (1988) three professional tasks of legitimation, research, and instruction. The notion that life processes could be normatively researched, legitimized identifiable departures from or delays in normal development as targets of intervention, and related to Foucault's (2008a) "grids of intelligibility." A developmental grid of intelligibility, to understand how life *should* be or normally proceed, legitimized psychologists' and counsellors' roles as arbiters and remediators of normality and abnormality. Messy human suffering or troubling abnormalities ("deviance") could be assessed against life's normalities, and remediated back to normal (see Rose 1990). Concepts like "arrested development" made their way far enough into the public consciousness (i.e. as looping effects) to serve as the name for a 1980s "hip-hop" band. Importantly for counsellor education, however, normative and developmentally oriented social science research helped to legitimize the earlier guidance-oriented work of counsellors, playing an important role in informing the knowledge and practices of counsellors-in-training. For example, one of the ACA's important professional publications remains the *Journal of Counseling and Development*, while the *British Journal of Guidance and Counselling* continues to be an important professional journal in the UK.

The kind of normative and developmental social science I have been describing is based on claims that may seem commonsensical, bringing normative social science into a hoped-for equivalence with the natural sciences (Gergen 1982). Scientific knowledge derived from the latter kind of science finds its applications in new technologies, and helps to engineer solutions to problems perplexing people. My initial exposure and fascination for psychology as a social science in the 1970s was partly based on a logic which appeals to many would-be counsellors seeking to be helpful by applying forms of psychological knowledge. Counsellors, by this logic (see Shean 2013), can acquire the "technology" (i.e. information, skills) to help people who suffer and lag behind norms and potentials to overcome such suffering and achieve their potentials. Basing counselling (and counsellor training) on such normative, developmentally oriented knowledge, enabled a scientific legitimacy and helpful promise that—like medicine—there was expertise by which one could diagnose concerns and intervene when people's lives went awry.

It helps to see the social and psychological sciences as engaging graduate students as future practitioner-researchers seeking to add to counselling's knowledge base. While developmental psychology shares some overlap with biomedical knowledge, where psychological knowledge and biomedical knowledge become almost orthogonal is around understandings of psychopathology (Insel and Cuthbert 2015). At the start of this chapter definitions of counselling speaks in some way to how counsellors help to enhance mental health, historically counsellors have not focused on concerns that would not be considered among the more severe forms of psychopathology. Clinical psychologists or psychiatrists are typically the professionals who diagnose and treat such psychopathology, or mental disorders (e.g. http://www.cpa.ca/aboutcpa/cpasections/clinicalpsychology/). On the front lines of service provision, however, counsellors are being asked to work with more serious mental health issues than ever before (e.g. Prince 2015), and to receive third-party payment they are often expected to see clients with more serious mental disorders (Weil 2015). Counsellors-in-training, in other words, can expect to face client needs that others would consider psychiatric in nature. While their training and graduate research opportunities generally do not fit the same patterns described earlier, these students often enter a mental health service culture where their ability to assess and respond to more serious mental health concerns can be important.

Stepping back a bit, an understandable yet informal and indirect relationship developed between the research and instruction occurring in graduate counsellor education programs, and the expert services required for public and private mental health. Competing versions of that expertise, leadership, and professionalism have coexisted since counselling's earliest days, playing out in different academic and "legislative" agendas (Buchanan 2003). These agendas become evident in turf wars between academics seeking to define practice through their research programs, professional association leadership roles, and involvement in government-appointed regulatory boards (see House 2004; Postle 2007). This is not to suggest that such academic leadership is odious or pursued without good intent, but professional developments, like those associated with medicalization, are incubated in and advocated from universities. Counsellor educators and graduate students working with them often develop and scientifically evaluate the interventions and approaches that become the instructable and accountable (i.e. evidence-based) practices required for front-line service (Bobbitt et al. 2012; O'Donohue and Maragakis 2016). They work to find ways to address emergent issues, such as maintaining professionalism despite reductions in mental health services (e.g. Acuff et al. 1999). However, another academic development has been to use critical theory and poststructuralist insights to draw attention to developments in practice which concern counsellors.

Postmodern and Poststructuralist Counselling?

Counselling today, in the eyes of one critic, may have shifted from a factory metaphor focused on developing and fixing people, to a postmodern metaphor focused on restoring people for participation in the marketplace (Kvale 2002). A "postmodern" approach to counselling also emerged in the 1980s and 1990s, while scientific "metanarratives" (Lyotard 1984) like those of developmental psychology (Burman 1994; Henriques et al. 1984; Morss 1996) became a critical target. A kind of essentialism had been implicit to psychology's modern social science, one based on the view that aspects of being human, such as being a woman (Bohan 1993) or describing humans concerns (Chalkley 2004), could be explained objectively, or "as they were." The related poststructuralist critique of this kind of psychological essentializing was premised on the discursive insights of Foucault (1968, 2008b), which came to play a role in the culture and social science "wars" of the 1990s (see Hacking 1999). The generative potentials of these postmodern and poststructuralist ideas were also finding their way into a range of new counselling approaches (Anderson 1997; De Shazer 1985; White and Epston 1990). Relatedly, there was an explosion of new qualitative methods of research associated with postmodern and poststructuralist approaches to the social sciences (Denzin and Lincoln 1994, 2000; Gubrium and Holstein 2007). Where modern research by psychologists was hitched to explaining the diagnosable and treatable essentials and abnormalities of human behavior, postmodern and poststructuralist critiques and practices seemed, for some, to be heading toward anarchy and illegitimacy (e.g. Held 1995).

I have engaged with both modern and postmodern worlds of practicing, learning, and teaching counselling—and this extends to participating in the science informing each world. After a preliminary exposure to constructivist thinking (e.g. Kelly 1963: Watzlawick et al. 1974) during my graduate schooldays (I completed a quantitative dissertation), new postmodern ideas of practice were becoming popular. My exposure to readings and workshops with therapist authors like Michael White (White and Epston 1990), Steve de Shazer (1985), and Harlene Anderson (1997) brought excitement, creativity, and teeth-gnashing over how to use these ideas and practices as a community mental health psychologist in a rural and remote location (see Strong 1993). For others, engaging with such ideas and practices (e.g. Weingarten 1991) brought a recognition of power and the situatedness of meaning/meaning-making—a recognition that also prompted tensions during my years of public and private practice. These tensions developed alongside growing expectations that I use what I have been describing as a medicalizing discourse of counselling: treatment for DSM-diagnosed disorders. Another therapist author had described working from such expectations as being like having "big brother in the consulting room" (Wylie 1994: 21). This concern continues to seem excessive, but it spoke to a very modern example of mentioned in this chapter's previous section counselling legislative agendas.

Counsellor education now technically subsumes both modern and postmodern approaches to practice (e.g. a popular theories textbook now includes a chapter on the "postmodern therapies," Corey 2016). It also continues to respect that pluralism and personal preference are priorities for counsellors as well as students when choosing approaches to practice (Cooper and McLeod 2011; Heinonen and Orlinksy 2013). Along with such a plurality of counselling approaches to learn are considerations given to issues of cultural inclusivity (Hays and Erford 2013) and social justice (Chung and Bemak 2012; Goodman and Gorski 2014). This latter curricular attention also departs from an essentializing and universalizing approach taken until recently in the modern psychological research, informing how counselling is to be learned and practiced (e.g. De Vos 2012; Stam 2015).

Boulder Model Training: EBP and PBE

Counselling psychologists, like their clinical psychologist colleagues, have championed the Boulder model for developing scientist practitioners, but there has been little consistency regarding how this model translates educationally or in practice (e.g. Ridley and Laird 2015). The scientist-practitioner model gained further importance in recent decades under the banner of EBP, with graduate students taking up roles in building the evidence base for different disorders and interventions, while also being expected to practice in evidence-based ways (see Chwalisz 2003; Rousseau and Gunia 2016).

The logic of EBP makes eminent sense against a historical backdrop of troubling mental health interventions that have included lobotomies, harmful medications, and electro-convulsive therapies. In this respect, EBP helps to remove unsafe practices from use, but where it comes up short for many practitioners is in how prescriptive and how decontextualized its presumptive use should be for actual practice. Some of the key debates (e.g. APA 2006; Borntrager et al. 2009; Smedslund 2016) have been over the extent to which mental health interventions can be standardized and prescribed as protocols, the generalizability of contextual considerations for their use, and perceived needs for treatment integrity. For educational purposes, EBP has become the "gold standard" training expectation, and this translates to a need for proficiency in following the standardized manuals and best practice guidelines associated with their use (Chwalisz 2003; Timmermans and Berg 2003). However, while the Boulder scientist-practitioner model of training may have helped to legitimize the profession and training of psychologists (and counsellors), important critics have seen its approach to science and practice as excessively medicalized (e.g. Albee 2000).

On the front lines of counselling there has also been a related push for PBE, a client- and outcome-informed approach based on client feedback, with respect to *their* goals in making client-sought differences (see Gabbay and le May 2011; Green and Latchford 2012; Wampold and Imel 2015). While EBP advocates prescribe using interventions in standardized ways, PBE flips things so that client feedback is used to inform how the counselling process would develop. One could see chicken and egg arguments for EBP and PBE, but becoming more rigorous and client-satisfying in one's practice can suggest at least two ways forward for the counsellor as scientist-practitioner: one being focused on knowing the psychological science for addressing generalized concerns, while the other focuses on hearing from clients how interventions are, in their eyes, making a difference—or not.

A medicalizing discourse of DSM-5 diagnoses, and evidence-based treatments to address diagnosed DSM-5 disorders, offers a structured way to instruct, supervise, and evaluate the learning and practice of graduate counsellors. For some this direction could bring science and practice into alignment, enabling the precision or accuracy expected from such training to be reflected in the judgments and practice of counsellors, (Miller et al. 2015; Spengler et al. 2009). Despite the medicalizing structure and training associated with it, this clinical science direction has only produced modest results, results the researchers put down to "overconfidence" and insufficient scientific rigor (Miller et al. 2015; Tackett et al. 2016). For some, such findings translate to a need to "double down" on expectations for trainee adherence to standardized practice (e.g. Southam-Gerow et al. 2016). For others, while training and client feedback might modestly improve outcome-related practices of trainees, such improvements might reflect "as good as it gets" (Owen et al. 2016). The training and supervision of counsellors has not measured up to expectation, despite greater clarity on a common language and approach to practice. From a recent survey of training directors in counselling psychology programs, the researchers concluded that "revisiting the very idea of the scientist–practitioner model" was essential (Ridley and Laird 2015: 261).

The literature I have been citing mostly reflects research of doctoral-level training and education in counselling psychology. Master's-level training programs in counselling most frequently are housed in the same departments as these doctoral programs (Jackson and Scheel 2013), and many Master's students transition into doctoral studies. The difference in expected competencies and curricula has sometimes set off tensions within and between accrediting bodies such as the American Psychological Association (for doctoral programs) and the Council of Accreditation of Counseling and Related Educational Programs (for Master's programs). As Lawson (2016) recently suggested, distinctive identity-forging efforts by psychologists are also occurring for professional counsellors who want to be understood by the public as offering something more than a less developed form of counselling psychologists' practice. At the start of this chapter definitions offered for counselling psychology and counselling helped to illustrate nuanced differences though one could be forgiven in seeing definitional overlaps.

Regardless of the professional identity differences, educators of counsellors and counselling psychologists have clear overlap in curricular foci and content. A recent review of articles focused on counsellor education highlighted that the counselling profession's efforts have largely concentrated on developing and evaluating new interventions, while giving less attention to pedagogical reflections and innovations (Barrio Minton et al. 2014). Another review of the counsellor education literature recently focused on professional competence and how to best address perceived deficiencies in students and training (Rust, Raskin, and Hill 2013). For many counsellor educators, answering such deficiencies requires training according to researcher-developed competency matrices (see Swank et al. 2012; Truax and Carkhuff 1967) akin to those used in medical training (Deveugele et al. 2005).

Clients have also played an increasing, yet general, training role in enhancing the practices of the counsellors they see—through the feedback they offer (Tracey et al. 2014). This kind of client feedback research has been somewhat helpful in refocusing counsellor training and supervision, to include more of a client-satisfaction orientation, a focus that has not always been consistent with accepted views of EBP (Laska et al. 2014; Minieri et al. 2015). This may be an argument worth heeding, for restoring a pedagogical focus on client-centeredness where a narrow technicism or methodolatry (see Hansen 2006; Martin et al. 2003) focused on discrete interventions (i.e. EBP) and competencies has dominated.

I have been describing issues that have preoccupied counsellor educators in recent decades. Some might see these differences as further evidence of a perennial debate between the artistic and scientific sides of the profession (e.g. Nystul 2016), over what should prevail in preparing graduate counsellors for work with clients. It is an issue that relates to how human concerns get discussed and addressed in counselling with respect to aspects of the human condition that only recently have been medicalized (Conrad 2007; Rapley et al. 2011).

Medicalizing Tensions in Counsellor Education?

Counsellors have been trying to reconcile their traditional notions of pluralistic and relationally oriented practice with medicalizing developments—like DSM and EBP—since the late 1990s. The obvious tensions arise out of the profession's humanistic and existential traditions focused on meaning and holistic well-being—people are more than potential vessels of pathology seeking proper diagnosis and treatment (Hansen 2003, 2014). However, other developments are shaping the art/science debates, such as an increased focus on client strengths and cultural inclusiveness (Tomlinson-Clarke and Georges 2014; Zalaquett et al. 2008). Modern/postmodern notions of practice also shape these debates as the former notion presumes scientific knowledge should be reliably applied when understanding and addressing human concerns (e.g. Gardner 2016; Shurts 2015). To present counselling's future otherwise is tantamount, for many moderns, to taking an anti-vaccination public health stance.

Another educational tension related to medicalizing discourse arises from how to train, supervise, and evaluate counsellors to square particular details of clients and their circumstances with generalized knowledge derived from psychological science. Central to this tension is how the experimental conditions yielding standardized protocols or manuals for using EBPs bear little resemblance to the immediacies and exigencies of front-line practice. Some see a translational need to focus supervisors on how to facilitate contextualizing such generalized EBP knowledge or competencies to particular client circumstances (Chang 2013; Miller et al. 2010). Another version of this competency-focused approach to training are "best practices" which tend to be less prescriptive in use than standardized EBP interventions (Hansen 2006; Thompson 2013). Regardless, over time trainees are expected to acquire and demonstrate capabilities to adapt "best" practices or EBPs to particular needs and circumstances of clients. A question can arise: to what extent are the EBPs or best practices adapted to clients, or clients adapted to the requirements of EBPs and best practices? The most common tension seen to accompany such contextualizing and translating of EBPs tends be over what this means for an EBP intervention's "treatment integrity" (Hagermoser Sanetti and Kratochwill 2014). In a student, supervisor, or practicing counsellors' thinking: when or how does an evidence-based treatment become invalidated? To what extent must competent practice be evaluated according to the scripts or protocols for EBP (Muse and McManus 2013)? Understandable anxieties arise for students who grapple with such tensions in their training and supervised practice (Daniels and Larson 2001).

The primary, evidence-supported focus of counsellor training and supervision relates to the student's capacity for developing and sustaining a good working alliance (WA) with clients (Knox and Cooper 2015; Norcross 2011; Wampold and Imel 2015). Students today need to develop ease in engaging with an increasingly diverse clientele. While a micro-skills focus that built on Carl Rogers' (1958) clinical writing launched this direction, Rogers' insights were based on a largely white, relatively affluent, clientele. Over time, it became hard to ignore social justice and cultural dimensions in the relationships that counsellors, and counsellors-in-training, need to forge with clients to be helpful (e.g. Tarvydas et al. 2015). An interim step in this direction came from Sue et al. (1992), who developed and advocated for "multicultural counseling competencies," to overcome a monocultural approach based on a presumed Caucasian and affluent clientele. While helping to shift the training of counsellors toward greater cultural responsiveness and inclusivity, it was a somewhat monolithic effort—focused beyond prior Caucasian-centric training, to *general* cultural sensitivities and competencies. As with Rogers' writing on enhancing relationships with clients, Sue, Arredondo, and McDavis' initial work also needed further nuancing and updating, to encompass an "intersectional" approach (Johnson and Munch 2009). "Intersectionality" refers to the multiple identity characteristics and "social locations" one may have; with some such characteristics/locations becoming more salient or relevant than others in the emerging conversational work of counselling.

A clunky version of intersectionality might be seen in a circumstance where a client's (or counsellor's) identities include such "locations" as woman, lesbian, Caribbean, unemployed, and single mother. Potentially, any one of these locations finds its salience or relevance to counselling should it be a source of concern or potential resilience. Some locations might be only tangentially related to the client's presenting concern, while other locations might be directly related. Suppose the above client's presenting concern is about an abusive teenage daughter?

Seeking to better address such complexities and intersectionalities brought me to a discursive approach to counselling (see Lock and Strong 2012) , for reasons related to concerns with medicalizing discourse. My concerns relate to distal and proximal influences vying for and shaping what gets possibly said and accomplished in the highly situated practice of counselling (see Gale et al. 2004; Strong 2016) . This last statement needs further unpacking since I have been primarily describing medicalizing discourse in "distal" ways typical to someone adopting a critical discourse perspective (e.g. Fairclough 1989, 1992). Discourse conversationally operates like one of those "locations" just described—as if in a generalized circumstance of fairly uniform meaning (a situated common sense or logic) and accustomed action. Where the tensions come up in educational and counselling conversations, relates to where medicalizing discourse is put to use; where it is supposed to guide those conversations. These are conversations where the salience or relevance of what is being discussed, for client and counsellor, is hardly static in how their conversation develops. Knowledge of the client's intersectional locations (as well as the counsellor's) can inform such fluid and highly situated conversations, but will not provide a stepwise regression analysis of what should be determining the conversation or its outcomes.

Supported by more rigorous science than that which is normal for discussing and evaluating other responses to human concerns (e.g. relationally, economically, spiritually), medicalizing discourse informs "governmentality" (Hook 2007) by seeming the expert way to address such concerns. It becomes a means for expertly helping others and oneself manage symptoms and chronic conditions to maintain an optimal quality of life (Madsen 2015). As a distal discourse, medicalization influences counselling and the training/supervisory relationship. Other discourses similarly have distal influences (e.g. social justice; neoliberal), but these do not promise the same, science-backed expertise one expects from medicalizing discourse.

Proximal aspects of counselling discourse were an initial research focus when I became a counsellor educator and related to my interest in the discursive (narrative, solution-focused, and collaborative) approaches to counselling (e.g. Strong 2002) . I took seriously the claim of the practitioner-authors developing these approaches (e.g. Anderson 1997): that in the conversational work of counselling clients and counsellors could construct and deconstruct concerns as clients experienced and understood them. This meant turning to a micro-focus acquainting me with the methodologically fastidious research of conversation analysts (e.g. Pain 2009; Ten Have 1999) and discursive psychologists (e.g. Edwards and Potter 1992). Important in these approaches is how turn-taking in conversation shapes what gets talked into significance. While larger cultural discourses (such as psychological discourse, see Edwards and Potter 1992) clearly have distal influences on dialogue, they don't determine what is said and accomplished by counsellor and client in face-to-face conversation. My interest was in sensitizing counsellors to their reflexive involvement in conversationally engaging clients in meaning-making processes, and that meant examining such things as conversational ethics (Strong and Sutherland 2007), conversational evidence (Strong et al. 2008), and even "wordsmithing" (Strong 2006). I wanted to show what was "constructed" (Strong and Pyle 2009) and deconstructed (Strong and Schultz 2010) in the conversational work of counselling, particularly for how that work occurred. I was interested in what clients and counsellors accomplished through their ways of conversing, and how that conversing was experienced.

The proximal aspect of counselling's conversational work tends to be learned as discrete skills, based on an information-transmission metaphor of communication (Lakoff and Johnson 1980; Turnbull 2003). Counsellor educators' variations on this metaphor focus on training students to demonstrate accurate communication micro-skills, best practices, and intervention and treatment protocols. At worst, students learn to preoccupy themselves with their responses and focus less on clients' communications. Maturana and Varela (1988) have mockingly referred to a related "tube metaphor," through which people purportedly should be able to "instructively interact." Conversation analysts and discursive psychologists, by contrast, see talk as a relational and communicative process as well as accomplishment—something done and built upon, or departed with each conversational turn (Pain 2009). It is in this sense that they and discursive counsellors consider talking as constructive (or deconstructive) while also being social.

These discursive (proximal and distal) views of counselling are only starting to find their way into counsellor education (e.g. Paré 2013) and can be perplexing for students as well as educators. Counselling by this view involves a conversational negotiation of how the counselling process develops. The discursive influences on how the client's concern is understood and responded to are also raised and reflected upon, while alternative discursive resources are collaboratively proposed and evaluated for their fit and utility in addressing the client's presenting concern. Such discursive resources are meanings and ways of communicating made accessible by alternative discourses, to avoid a single discourse totalizing the conversational work or outcome. Bereavement has offered an example, where a singular medicalizing discourse leaves out other discourses (e.g. spiritual, financial, relational) from which clients might want to discuss their experiences (e.g. Frances 2013). Expert medicalizing conversations tend to standardize diagnostic and treatment details the medical expert needs through information exchanges spelled out in manualized conversational protocols. For students of counselling, these protocols can be reassuring, offering expected and standardized conversational protocols to guide the conversation; a discursive and negotiated approach to counselling is more ambiguous relationally and situationally speaking.

Medicalizing discourse in counselling and counsellor education presents a challenge for counsellors and counsellors-in-training who take up relational, meaning-focused, culturally inclusive, feminist, and other approaches to (or discourses of) counselling. This is where the pluralistic traditions of counselling sometimes run headlong into the standardized expectations associated with the medicalizing discourse of DSM-5 diagnoses and EBPs. Counsellor education programs tend to teach from curricula based on pluralistic approaches to, or discourses of, practice. Typically, it is in courses like assessment or interventions, where DSM-5 diagnoses and evidence-based interventions are taught, that medicalizing discourse can run counter to that pluralism. While counsellor education websites highlight student learning of both medicalized and pluralistic discourses, it is in their practice that students can find medicalizing tensions of greatest relevance for their learning and practice (Strong et al. 2015). Graduates from counsellor education programs tend to use varied discourses of practice, despite having to justify their work using medicalizing discourse which can produce tensions for them (Strong et al. 2012).

Coda

Medicalizing discourse has arguably provided mental health professionals with a common language for understanding and responding to clients' presenting concerns. However, counsellors and students of counselling have traditionally approached client concerns using discourses of practice that can supplement or, at worst, be at odds with a standardized medicalizing discourse. With good reason readers would cringe at the thought of a postmodern or discursively oriented neurosurgeon, but counsellors are not doing conversational equivalents of surgery with clients. While considerable research has gone into identifying treatment effects of different interventions and practices, qualities of the conversational relationship are consistently evaluated by clients as most helpful. Conversational work in counselling and counsellor education can involve a negotiation of discursive resources (medicalizing discourse included) that can be reflected upon and judiciously taken up. Discursive awareness and resourcefulness in good conversational relationships is important not only to counsellors, but to counsellor educators, students, and the clients they aim to best serve.

References

Abbott, A. (1988). *The system of professions: An essay on the division of expert labor*. Chicago: University of Chicago Press.

Acuff, C., Bennett, B. E., Bricklin, P. M., Canter, M. B., Knapp, S. J., Moldawsky, S., et al. (1999). Considerations for ethical practice in managed care. *Professional Psychology, Research and Practice, 30*(6), 563–575.

Albee, G. W. (2000). The boulder model's fatal flaw. *American Psychologist, 55*(2), 247–248.

Anderson, H. (1997). *Conversation, language, and possibilities: A postmodern approach to therapy*. New York: Basic Books.

APA Presidential Task Force on Evidence-Based Practice and American Psychological Association. (2006). Evidence-based practice in psychology. *American Psychologist, 61*(4), 271–285.

Barrio Minton, C. A., Wachter Morris, C. A., & Yaites, L. D. (2014). Pedagogy in counselor education: A 10-year content analysis of journals. *Counselor Education and Supervision, 53*(3), 162–177.

Berman, J. S., & Norton, N. C. (1985). Does professional training make a therapist more effective? *Psychological Bulletin, 98*(2), 401–407.

Binet, A. S. T. (1916). *The development of intelligence in children: The binet-simon scale* (E. S. Kite, Trans.), Publications of the training school at Vineland New Jersey department of research No. 11. Baltimore: Williams & Wilkins.

Bobbitt, B. L., Cate, R. A., Beardsley, S. D., Azocar, F., & McCulloch, J. (2012). Quality improvement and outcomes in the future of professional psychology: Opportunities and challenges. *Professional Psychology, Research and Practice, 43*(6), 551–559.

Bohan, J. S. (1993). Regarding gender: Essentialism, constructionism, and feminist psychology. *Psychology of Women Quarterly, 17*(1), 5–21.

Boorse, C. (1977). Health as a theoretical concept. *Philosophy of Science, 44*(4), 542–573.

Borntrager, C. F., Chorpita, B. F., Higa-McMillan, C., & Weisz, J. R. (2009). Provider attitudes toward evidence-based practices: Are the concerns with the evidence or with the manuals? *Psychiatric Services (Washington, D.C.), 60*(5), 677–681.

Buchanan, R. (2003). Legislative warriors: American psychiatrists, psychologists, and competing claims over psychotherapy in the 1950s. *Journal of the History of the Behavioral Sciences, 39*(3), 225–249.

Burman, E. (1994). *Deconstructing developmental psychology*. London: Routledge.
Carkhuff, R. R. (1967). Toward a comprehensive model of facilitative interpersonal processes. *Journal of Counseling Psychology, 14*(1), 67–72.
Carter, E. A., & McGoldrick, M. (Eds.). (1980). *The changing family life cycle: A framework for family therapy*. New York: Gardner Press.
Chalkley, A. J. (2004). The description of concerns. *Psychology and Psychotherapy, 77*(2), 207–230.
Chang, J. (2013). A contextual-functional meta-framework for counselling supervision. *International Journal for the Advancement of Counselling, 35*(2), 71–87.
Chung, R. C., & Bemak, F. (2012). *Social justice counseling: The next steps beyond multiculturalism*. Thousand Oaks, CA: Sage Publications.
Chwalisz, K. (2003). Evidence-based practice: A framework for twenty-first century scientist-practitioner training. *The Counseling Psychologist, 31*(5), 497–528.
Conrad, P. (2007). *The medicalization of society*. Baltimore: Johns Hopkins University Press.
Cooper, M., & McLeod, J. (2011). *Pluralistic counselling and psychotherapy*. Thousand Oaks, CA: Sage.
Corey, G. (2016). *Theory and practice of counseling and psychotherapy* (10th ed.). Boston: Cengage Learning.
Corsini, R. J., & Wedding, D. (2010). *Current psychotherapies* (9th ed.). Belmont, CA: Brooks/Cole.
Cottle, W. C. (1953). Personal characteristics of counselors: I. *Personnel and Guidance Journal, 31*(7), 445–450.
Cox, R. D. (1945). *Counselors and their work*. Harrisburg, PA: Archives Press.
Daniels, J. A. (2001). Managed care, ethics, and counseling. *Journal of Counseling & Development, 79*(1), 119–122.
De Shazer, S. (1985). *Keys to solution in brief therapy*. New York: W.W. Norton.
De Vos, J. (2012). *Psychologisation in times of globalisation*. London: Routledge.
Denzin, N. K., & Lincoln, Y. S. (Eds.). (1994). *Handbook of qualitative research*. Thousand Oaks, CA: Sage.
Denzin, N. K., & Lincoln, Y. S. (Eds.). (2000). *Handbook of qualitative research* (2nd ed.). Thousand Oaks, CA: Sage.
Deveugele, M., Derese, A., Maesschalck, S. D., Willems, S., Driel, M. V., & Maeseneer, J. D. (2005). Teaching communication skills to medical students, a challenge in the curriculum? *Patient Education and Counseling, 58*(3), 265–270.

Duncan, B. L., Miller, S. D., Wampold, B. E., & Hubble, M. A. (Eds.). (2010). *The heart and soul of change: Delivering what works in therapy* (2nd ed.). Washington: American Psychological Association.

Durlak, J. A. (1979). Comparative effectiveness of paraprofessional and professional helpers. *Psychological Bulletin, 86*(1), 80–92.

Edwards, D., & Potter, J. (1992). *Discursive psychology*. London: Sage.

Erickson, F., & Shultz, J. J. (1982). *The counselor as gatekeeper: Social interaction in interviews*. New York: Academic Press.

Fairclough, N. (1989). *Language and power*. Harlow: Longman.

Fairclough, N. (1992). *Discourse and social change*. Cambridge: Polity Press.

Foster, J. M., Leppma, M., & Hutchinson, T. S. (2014). Students' perspectives on gatekeeping in counselor education: A case study. *Counselor Education and Supervision, 53*(3), 190–203.

Foucault, M. (1968). *Madness and civilization: A history of insanity in the age of reason* (R. Howard, Trans). New York: Vintage.

Foucault, M. (2008a). *The birth of biopolitics: Lectures at the collège de France, 1978–1979*. New York: Palgrave Macmillan.

Foucault, M. (2008b). *History of madness*. New York: Routledge.

Frances, A. (2013). *Saving normal: An insider's revolt against out-of-control psychiatric diagnosis, DSM-5, big pharma, and the medicalization of ordinary life*. New York: William Morrow.

Gabbay, J., & le May, A. (2011). *Practice-based evidence for healthcare: Clinical mindlines*. London: Routledge.

Gale, J., Lawless, J., & Roulston, K. (2004). Discursive approaches to clinical research. In T. Strong & D. Paré (Eds.), *Furthering talk: Advances in the discursive therapies* (pp. 125–144). New York: Kluwer Academic/Plenum.

Gardner, L. (2016). Metamodernism: A new philosophical approach to counseling. *Journal of Humanistic Counseling, 55*(2), 86–98.

Gergen, K. J. (1982). *Toward transformation in social knowledge*. New York: Springer-Verlag.

Goodman, D. M. (2016). The McDonaldization of psychotherapy: Processed foods, processed therapies, and economic class. *Theory & Psychology, 26*(1), 77–95.

Goodman, R. D., & Gorski, P. C. (Eds.). (2014). *Decolonizing "multicultural" counseling through social justice*. New York: Springer.

Green, D., & Latchford, G. (2012). *Maximising the benefits of psychotherapy: A practice-based evidence approach*. West Sussex: Wiley-Blackwell.

Hacking, I. (1999). *The social construction of what?* Cambridge, MA: Harvard University Press.

Hagermoser Sanetti, L. M., & Kratochwill, T. R. (Eds.). (2014). *Treatment integrity: A foundation for evidence-based practice in applied psychology*. Washington: American Psychological Association.

Hansen, J. T. (2003). Including diagnostic training in counseling curricula: Implications for professional identity development. *Counselor Education and Supervision, 43*(2), 96–107.

Hansen, J. T. (2006). Is the best practices movement consistent with the values of the counseling profession? A critical analysis of best practices ideology. *Counseling and Values, 50*(2), 154–161.

Hansen, J. T. (2014). Talking about counseling: A plea to return to humanistic language. *Journal of Humanistic Counseling, 53*(1), 22–33.

Hathaway, S. R. (1948). Some considerations relative to nondirective counseling as therapy. *Journal of Clinical Psychology, 4*, 226–231.

Hays, D. G., & Erford, B. T. (2013). *Developing multicultural counseling competence: A systems approach* (2nd ed.). Toronto, ON: Pearson Canada.

Heatherington, L., Messer, S. B., Angus, L., Strauman, T. J., Friedlander, M. L., & Kolden, G. G. (2012). The narrowing of theoretical orientations in clinical psychology doctoral training. *Clinical Psychology: Science and Practice, 19*(4), 364–374.

Heinonen, E., & Orlinsky, D. E. (2013). Psychotherapists' personal identities, theoretical orientations, and professional relationships: Elective affinity and role adjustment as modes of congruence. *Psychotherapy Research: Journal of the Society for Psychotherapy Research, 23*(6), 718–731.

Held, B. (1995). *Back to reality: A critique of postmodern theory in psychotherapy*. New York: W.W. Norton.

Henriques, J., Hollway, W., Urwin, C., Venn, C., & Walkerdine, V. (Eds.). (1984). *Changing the subject: Psychology, social regulation and subjectivity*. London: Methuen.

Holstein, J. A., & Gubrium, J. F. (Eds.). (2007). *Handbook of constructionist research*. New York: Guilford Press.

Hook, D. (2007). *Foucault, psychology and the analytics of power*. London: Palgrave Macmillan.

House, R. (2004). *Therapy beyond modernity: Deconstructing and transcending profession-centred therapy*. London: Karnac.

Hoyt, K. B. (1962). Guidance: A constellation of services. *Personnel and Guidance Journal, 40*(8), 690–697.

Insel, T. R., & Cuthbert, B. N. (2015). Brain disorders? Precisely. *Science, 348*(6234), 499–500.

Ivey, A. E., Ivey, M. B., & Simek-Morgan, L. (1993). *Counseling and psychotherapy: Integrating skills, theory, and practice* (3rd ed.). Englewood Cliffs, NJ: Prentice Hall.

Jackson, M. A., & Scheel, M. J. (2013). Quality of master's education: A concern for counseling psychology? *The Counseling Psychologist, 41*(5), 669–699.

Johnson, Y. M., & Munch, S. (2009). Fundamental contradictions in cultural competence. *Social Work, 54*(3), 220–231.

Kelly, G. A. (1963). *A theory of personality: The psychology of personal constructs*. New York: W.W. Norton.

Knox, R., & Cooper, M. (2015). *The therapeutic relationship in counselling and psychotherapy*. London: SAGE.

Kvale, S. (2002). The church, the factory and the market as metaphors for psychology. In C. V. Hofstein & L. Bäckman (Eds.), *Psychology at the turn of the millennium*, Vol. 2: *Social, developmental and clinical perspectives* (pp. 409–436). New York: Taylor & Francis.

Lakoff, G., & Johnson, M. (1980). *Metaphors we live by*. Chicago: University of Chicago Press.

Laska, K. M., Gurman, A. S., & Wampold, B. E. (2014). Expanding the lens of evidence-based practice in psychotherapy: A common factors perspective. *Psychotherapy (Chicago, Ill.), 51*(4), 467–481.

Lawson, G. (2016). On being a profession: A historical perspective on counselor licensure and accreditation. *Journal of Counselor Leadership and Advocacy, 3*(2), 71–84.

Lock, A., & Strong, T. (Eds.). (2012). *Discursive perspectives in therapeutic practice*. New York: Oxford University Press.

Lyotard, J. F. (1984). *The postmodern condition: A report on knowledge*. Minneapolis: University of Minnesota Press.

Madsen, O. J. (2015). Psychotherapists: Agents of change or maintenance men? In I. Parker (Ed.), *Handbook of Critical Psychology* (pp. 222–230). London: Routledge.

Mallinckrodt, B., & Nelson, M. L. (1991). Counselor training level and the formation of the psychotherapeutic working alliance. *Journal of Counseling Psychology, 38*(2), 133–138.

Martin, J., Sugarman, J., & Thompson, J. (2003). *Psychology and the question of agency*. Albany: State University of New York Press.

Maturana, H., & Varela, F. (1988). *The tree of knowledge: The biological roots of human understanding*. Boston: Shambhala.
Menne, J.M. (1975). A comprehensive set of counselor competencies. *Journal of Counseling Psychology, 22*(6), 547–553.
Miller, J. K., Todahl, J. L., & Platt, J. J. (2010). The core competency movement in marriage and family therapy: Key considerations from other disciplines. *Journal of Marital and Family Therapy, 36*(1), 59–70.
Miller, D. J., Spengler, E. S., & Spengler, P. M. (2015). A meta-analysis of confidence and judgment accuracy in clinical decision making. *Journal of Counseling Psychology, 62*(4), 553–567.
Minieri, A. M., Reese, R. J., Miserocchi, K. M., & Pascale-Hague, D. (2015). Using client feedback in training of future counseling psychologists: An evidence-based and social justice practice. *Counselling Psychology Quarterly, 28*(3), 305–323.
Morss, J. R. (1996). *Growing critical: Alternatives to developmental psychology*. London: Routledge.
Muse, K., & McManus, F. (2013). A systematic review of methods for assessing competence in cognitive-behavioural therapy. *Clinical Psychology Review, 33*(3), 484–499.
Neuer Colburn, A. A., Grothaus, T., Hays, D. G., & Milliken, T. (2016). A delphi study and initial validation of counselor supervision competencies. *Counselor Education and Supervision, 55*(1), 2–15.
Norcross, J. C. (Ed.). (2011). *Psychotherapy relationships that work: Evidence-based responsiveness* (2nd ed.). New York: Oxford University Press.
Nystul, M. S. (2016). *Introduction to counseling: An art and science perspective* (5th ed.). Los Angeles: SAGE.
O'Donohue, W., & Maragakis, A. (Eds.). (2016). *Quality improvement in behavioral health*. New York: Springer.
Ogunfowora, B., & Drapeau, M. (2008). Comparing counselling and clinical psychology professionals: Similarities and differences on theoretical orientations revisited. *International Journal for the Advancement of Counselling, 30*(2), 93–103.
Owen, J., Wampold, B. E., Kopta, M., Rousmaniere, T., & Miller, S. D. (2016). As good as it gets? Therapy outcomes of trainees over time. *Journal of Counseling Psychology, 63*(1), 12–19.
Pain, J. (2009). *Not just talking: Conversational analysis, harvey sacks' gift to therapy*. London: Karnac.
Paré, D. (2013). *The practice of collaborative counseling and psychotherapy: Developing skills in culturally mindful helping*. Los Angeles: Sage.

Postle, D. (2007). *Regulating the psychological therapies: From taxonomy to taxidermy* (2nd ed.). Ross-on-Wye: PCCS Books.

Prince, J. P. (2015). University student counseling and mental health in the United States: Trends and challenges. *Mental Health & Prevention, 3*(1–2), 5–10.

Rapley, M., Moncrieff, J., & Dillon, J. (2011). *De-Medicalizing misery: Psychiatry, psychology and the human condition*. New York: Palgrave Macmillan.

Ridley, C., & Laird, V. (2015). The scientist-practitioner model in counseling psychology programs: A survey of training directors. *Counselling Psychology Quarterly, 28*(3), 235–263.

Rogers, C. (1941). *Counseling and psychotherapy: Newer concepts in practice*. New York: Houghton Mifflin.

Rogers, C. (1958). The characteristics of a helping relationship. *Personnel and Guidance Journal, 37*(1), 6–16.

Rogers, C. (1973). Some new challenges. *American Psychologist, 28*(5), 379–387.

Rose, N. (1990). *Governing the soul: The shaping of the private self.* New York: Routledge.

Rousseau, D. M., & Gunia, B. C. (2016). Evidence-based practice: The psychology of EBP implementation. *Annual Review of Psychology, 67*(1), 667–692.

Rust, J. P., Raskin, J. D., & Hill, M. S. (2013). Problems of professional competence among counselor trainees: Programmatic issues and guidelines. *Counselor Education and Supervision, 52*(1), 30–42.

Shean, G. D. (2013). Controversies in psychotherapy research: Epistemic differences in assumptions about human psychology. *American Journal of Psychotherapy, 67*(1), 73–87.

Shurts, W. M. (2015). Infusing postmodernism into counseling supervision: Challenges and recommendations. *Journal of Counselor Preparation and Supervision, 7*(3), 11–132.

Smedslund, J. (2016). Practicing psychology without an empirical evidence-base: The bricoleur model. *New Ideas in Psychology, 43,* 50–56.

Southam-Gerow, M. A., McLeod, B. D., Arnold, C. C., et al. (2016). Initial development of a treatment adherence measure for cognitive-behavioral therapy for child anxiety. *Psychological Assessment, 28*(1), 70–80.

Spengler, P. M., White, M. J., Ægisdóttir, S., et al. (2009). The meta-analysis of clinical judgment project: Effects of experience on judgment accuracy. *The Counseling Psychologist, 37*(3), 350–399.

Stam, H. J. (2015). The historical boundedness of psychological knowledge and the ethics of shared understandings. *Journal of Theoretical and Philosophical Psychology, 35*(2), 117–127.
Strong, T. (1993). DSM-IV and describing problems in family therapy. *Family Process, 32,* 249–253.
Strong, T. (2002). Collaborative 'expertise' after the discursive turn. *Journal of Psychotherapy Integration, 12*(2), 218–232.
Strong, T. (2006). Wordsmithing in counselling? *European Journal of Psychotherapy and Counselling, 8*(3), 251–268.
Strong, T. (2016). Discursive awareness and resourcefulness: Bringing discursive researchers into closer dialogue with discursive therapists? In M. O'Reilly & J. Lester (Eds.), *Adult mental health: Discourse and conversation studies*. London: Palgrave Macmillan.
Strong, T., & Pyle, N. R. (2009). Constructing a conversational 'miracle': Examining the 'miracle question' as it is used in therapeutic dialogue. *Journal of Constructivist Psychology, 22*(4), 328–353.
Strong, T., & Schultz, L. (2010). Asking and answering deconstruction questions from within counselling dialogues. In J. Raskin, S. Bridges, & R. Neimeyer (Eds.), *Studies in meaning 4: Constructivist perspectives on theory, practice, and social justice* (pp. 123–150). New York: Pace University Press.
Strong, T., & Sutherland, O. A. (2007). Conversational ethics in psychological dialogues: Discursive and collaborative considerations. *Canadian Psychology, 48*(2), 94–105.
Strong, T., Busch, R. S., & Couture, S. (2008). Conversational evidence in therapeutic dialogue. *Journal of Marital and Family Therapy, 34*(3), 288–305.
Strong, T., Gaete, J., Sametband, I. N., French, J., & Eeson, J. (2012). Counsellors respond to the DSM-IV-TR. *Canadian Journal of Counselling and Psychotherapy, 46*(2), 85–106.
Strong, T., Ross, K. H., & Sesma-Vazquez, M. (2015). Counselling the (self?) diagnosed client: Generative and reflective conversations. *British Journal of Guidance and Counselling, 43*(5), 598–610.
Strong, T., Chondros, K., Job, C., & Vegter, V. (2017). Medicalizing Developments in Counsellor Education? Counselling and Counselling Psychology Students' Views. *Canadian Journal of Counselling and Psychotherapy, 57*, 161–186.
Strong, T., Chondros, K., Vegter, V., & Job, C. (forthcoming-b). Medicalizing tensions in counsellor education? European Journal of Psychotherapy and Counselling.

Sue, D. W., Arredondo, P., & McDavis, R. J. (1992). Multicultural counseling competencies and standards: A call to the profession. *Journal of Multicultural Counseling and Development, 20*(2), 64–88.
Super, D. E. (1953). A theory of vocational development. *American psychologist, 8*(5), 185–190.
Swank, J. M., Lambie, G. W., & Witta, E. L. (2012). An exploratory investigation of the counseling competencies scale: A measure of counseling skills, dispositions, and behaviors. *Counselor Education and Supervision, 51*(3), 189–206.
Tackett, J. L., Lilienfeld, S. O., Patrick, C. J., et al. (2016). It's time to broaden the replicability conversation: Thoughts for and from clinical psychological science. preprint for *Perspectives on Psychological Science*. Accessed December 29, 2016, from https://osf.io/preprints/psyarxiv/uwus7.
Tarvydas, V., Vazquez-Ramos, R., & Estrada-Hernandez, N. (2015). Applied participatory ethics: Bridging the social justice chasm between counselor and client. *Counseling and Values, 60*(2), 218–233.
Ten Have, P. (1999). *Doing conversation analysis: A practical guide*. Thousand Oaks, CA: Sage.
Thompson, R. A. (2013). *Professional school counseling: Best practices for working in the schools*. New York: Routledge.
Timmermans, S., & Berg, M. (2003). *The gold standard: The challenge of evidence-based medicine and standardization in health care*. Philadelphia: Temple University Press.
Tomlinson-Clarke, S. M., & Georges, C. M. (2014). DSM-5: A commentary on integrating multicultural and strength-based considerations into counseling training and practice. *The Professional Counselor, 4*(3), 272–281.
Tracey, T. J. G., Wampold, B. E., Lichtenberg, J. W., & Goodyear, R. K. (2014). Expertise in psychotherapy: An elusive goal? *The American Psychologist, 69*(3), 218–229.
Truax, C. B., & Carkhuff, R. (1967). *Toward effective counseling and psychotherapy: Training and practice*. Chicago: Aldine.
Tschacher, W., Junghan, U. M., & Pfammatter, M. (2014). Towards a taxonomy of common factors in psychotherapy: Results of an expert survey. *Clinical Psychology & Psychotherapy, 21*(1), 82–96.
Turnbull, W. (2003). *Language in action: Psychological models of conversation*. New York: Psychology Press.
Tyler, L. E. (1953). *The work of the counselor*. New York: Appleton-Century Crofts.
Wampold, B. E., & Imel, Z. E. (2015). *The great psychotherapy debate: The evidence for what makes psychotherapy work*. New York: Routledge.

Wampold, B. E., Flückiger, C., Del Re, A. C., et al. (2017). In pursuit of truth: A critical examination of meta-analyses of cognitive behavior therapy. *Psychotherapy Research, 27*(1), 14–32.
Watzlawick, P., Weakland, J., & Fisch, R. (1974). *Change: Principles of problem formation and problem resolution*. New York: W.W. Norton.
Weil, T. P. (2015). Insufficient dollars and qualified personnel to meet United States mental health needs. *Journal of Nervous and Mental Disease, 203*(4), 233–240.
Weingarten, K. (1991). The discourses of intimacy: Adding a social constructionist and feminist view. *Family Process, 30*(3), 285–305.
White, M., & Epston, D. (1990). *Narrative means to therapeutic ends*. New York: W.W. Norton.
Worden, J. W. (1991). *Grief counseling and grief therapy* (2nd ed.). New York: Springer.
Wright, H. W., & Darley, J. G. (1947). Counseling and guidance. *Journal of Educational Research, 41*(2), 116–125.
Wylie, M. S. (1994). Endangered species. *Family Therapy Networker, 18*(2), 20–33.
Zalaquett, C. P., Fuerth, K. M., Stein, C., Ivey, A. E., & Ivey, M. B. (2008). Reframing the DSM-IV-TR from a multicultural/social justice perspective. *Journal of Counseling & Development, 86*(3), 364–371.

10

Living with Tensions Associated with Medicalizing Counselling

To treat expertise as real and substantive is to treat it as something other than relational.
(Collins and Evans 2009: 2)

Conversation, then, is not merely a prelude to action, it is its very essence.
(Flores 2012: 5)

Part of the motivation for writing this book has been a concern for the future of an important conversational and relational practice: counselling. The critique of medicalization offered throughout this book should therefore be understood with respect to concerns about its dominance within a profession traditionally home to many discourses of practice (Cooper and McLeod 2011). As a discourse, like other discourses, medicalization affords certain meaningful resources and possibilities while constraining others, so this book should be read in that light. Counselling is a relationally oriented profession, making discourses—languages, how they get shared and reflected upon—central to what occurs in its conversational work with clients. What I have been describing as medicalizing tensions relate to concerns about potentially resourceful conversations of

T. Strong, *Medicalizing Counselling*, Palgrave Studies in the Theory and History of Psychology, DOI 10.1007/978-3-319-56699-3_10

counselling being constrained by requirements associated with medicalizing discourse's diagnose-and-treat logic and language (Conrad 2007).

Charles Taylor (1985) has described humans as "self-interpreting animals" who do not find the language for self-determination on their own. This observation takes on added importance when considering the quality of our emotional lives and value-based judgments—the grist for a lot of what people seek from counselling. The emotionally neutral and purportedly value-free assumptions and medicalizing language of health and psychological science may be helpful to counselling in ways worth supplementing or navigating around. For the historian of psychology, Kurt Danziger (1997: 192): "The more uncompromising psychologists became in their exclusive commitment to the requirements of scientific language the more impoverished their descriptions became, at least from the point of view of ordinary usage." Quite understandably, medicalizing incorporated psychological discourse into its discourse of expertise is also taken up by the public in identity-shaping and service-expecting ways before counsellors even sit down with clients. It is a discourse of convenience for administrators seeking a way to ration counselling as a mental health service (e.g. Motes and Smith 2014). However, supplementing or navigating around medicalizing discourse is problematic for those who require services on counselling's front lines to be delivered in ways consistent with how they were evaluated in experimentally controlled conditions (e.g. Proctor et al. 2009).

As we have explored throughout this book, some medicalizing tensions, for counsellors, arise from differences over communication or language use metaphors (see Lakoff and Johnson 1980; Turnbull 2003). What is supposed to take place in counselling's conversations? The answer, if you are a medical professional, is a highly focused exchange of information relevant for making a proper diagnosis, and expertly delivering an intervention, an exchange central to EBP. The informational value of the language reliably used purportedly makes medicalizing discourse in counselling effective, though other details salient or relevant to the client or counsellor may go undiscussed. Acquiring such deliverable psychological and medical information has been central to building the knowledge or evidence base of mental health service delivery. However, the information shifts over time. Diagnoses come and go (Cushman

1995; Jutel 2011), with even whole classification systems like the DSM-5 discredited in the eyes of some experts (e.g. Frances 2013; Insel 2013). For Ian Hacking (1995), some of the issues come with researching, then treating, "human kinds" as if they were "natural kinds."

Humans, of course, cannot be understood like rocks and trees; they are, as Bruno Latour (1996) has suggested, interpreting animals who can object to how they are being objectified. In some forms of counselling such objections might be understood as resistance, traceable to different metaphors of communication. As a discursive activity, counselling involves more than information exchanges and expertly delivered directives; it can be where discourse differences are expected, even welcomed (Paré 2013), for how they are reflexively produced in counselling's conversational work. Counselling involves clients and counsellors talking and listening in constructive as well as deconstructive ways; if not, they are probably keeping things the same (Kozart 2002). Medicalizing tensions arise over what a medicalizing discourse of counselling leaves out as irrelevant to the conversational work of counselling.

There can be a mechanistic aspect to medicalizing discourse when practice is reduced to protocols that link experimental science, mental health administration, and front-line practice. Such protocols and the information that enables them are developed from normative social science which treats particular interactions as generalizable formal knowledge that elsewhere inform an algorithmic approach to AI (Chun 2011, 2016; Steiner 2012). This is an approach based on standardizing how problems and interventions should be both understood and acted upon (Bowker and Star 2000; Busch 2011) Standardizing counselling has been a legitimizing move taken up as informing EBP in psychology and counselling psychology (Chwalisz 2003; Dozois 2013). The intentions behind this direction for practice were good (that people should get safe and effective interventions) but tend to hold practice to a single medicalizing discourse. Symptom relief is seldom the only reason clients come for counselling.

Centuries ago, the philologist Vico ([1744] 2001) wrote of a need that ran counter to the essentializing project of Enlightenment philosophy and modern science. The challenge Vico saw was one of *linguistic poverty* when the available terms for making sense of human experience were inadequate. Needed, he wrote, was poetic wisdom to address such places where words come up short for people, institutions, and nations. Medicalizing discourse sometimes begs supplementation and critical reflection in counselling. Many counsellors use approaches where reflexive meaning-making is central, and that translates to seeing meanings for client concerns as fluid, while the interventions to address "those concerns" require some element of customization to circumstance and preference. Meanings, in this sense, are not standardizable, despite persistent psychological efforts to make them so (De Vos 2012). While counsellors talked, in still essentializing ways, of constructively "reframing" client meanings for decades (e.g. Frankl 2006; Watzlawick et al. 1974), poststructural approaches to meaning developed in linguistic philosophy (e.g. Wittgenstein 1953) and within the philosophy of science (Hacking 1983). Put simply, this revolution in meaning highlighted that the words we (scientists' included—there are no meanings for things "as they are") put to experience were ours, what matters is how effective they are when put to use (Rorty 1989).

Critical scholars like Foucault also took up these insights to examine how madness (2008) and psychiatric power (2006) were socially constructed over time, particularly for the reflexive effects of these constructions in governing peoples' lives. New counselling approaches were relatedly developed from these insights into critically informed, reflexive language use, and became the basis for the discursive approaches to counselling: narrative, solution-focused, and collaborative (e.g. Friedman 1993; Lock and Strong 2012). Where medicalizing tensions really come to roost for this latter group of counsellors is over essentializing and standardizing expert meanings for client concerns as medical or psychiatric diagnoses.

While trained to screen for symptoms of psychiatric concern, the focus of most counsellors tends to be on addressing concerns that would be normally considered non-psychiatric in nature, to address difficulties or problems in living (Aubrey 1983; Szasz 1961; Tyler 1953). Their clientele has typically been those whose difficulties or problems might be accompanied by low degrees of anxiety or depression—the "worried well" (Miller et al. 1988). There has, however, been some fluidity to the meaning of this phrase that has generated concern. Specifically, the symptom severity levels for clinically differentiating sadness from depression (Horwitz and Wakefield 2007) or fear from anxiety (Horwitz and Wakefield 2012) have been changing in medicalizing ways. Critics of this expansion of formerly normal aspects of the human condition into diagnosable disorders usually cite a "Big Pharma" influence at work (e.g. Rapley et al. 2011; Whitaker and Cosgrove 2015). However, these medicalizing effects don't stop at diagnosing more psychiatric conditions or treating them with more medications, they cross over to constrain the meanings and dialogues of counselling as well.

Medicalizing Conversational Possibilities?

For some years, I have critiqued what I have been calling medicalizing tensions (e.g. Strong 1993, 1995), beginning initially as a counselling psychologist in public practice, up until my current role as a counsellor educator at a large Canadian university (Strong and Sesma-Vazquez 2015). I have been concerned about what is left out of medicalizing discourse, or the implications of medicalizing discourse when it has the potential to dominate or constrain the practices and education of counsellors. Over these years, I have heard a range of views about the DSMIV and DSM-5, and the EBPs that should be used to treat DSM-diagnosed disorders. Perhaps the most frequently expressed view is that counsellors should get on with providing evidence for their own practices (i.e. on DSM terms); or, by pushing for diagnoses for concerns they address in their practice that are currently not deemed compensable for counsellors, addressing those concerns. Why not medicalize relational concerns, so that treatment for relational concerns would become reimbursable, was one debate I was invited into (Strong 2015; Wamboldt et al. 2015). My concern has been fairly consistent over the years: to diagnose something as treatable initiates both an essentializing and a constraining (or standardizing) process related to aspects of what I have been calling medicalizing tensions.

There has been a particular modern view of professions that can be seen to accompany this kind of essentializing and standardizing of practice (Abbott 1988): that professions are gatekeepers for serving others on the basis of particular kinds of knowledge and expertise. Susskind and Susskind (2015) recently referred to this gatekeeping as a kind of "grand bargain" with society, and rhetorically posed the question: "to what problem are the professions our solution?" (2015: 38–39). Answering their question, with "mental health problems" is how medicalizing discourse paints counsellors into a professional corner of sorts, a corner in which they are clearly professional subordinates, and where a prospective clientele is also inside the gate often using the same discourse to understand and govern themselves (Hook 2007; Illouz 2008). Susskind and Susskind (2015: 139) later went on to write: "In the professions, as elsewhere, the corner shop will be displaced by the supermarket, bringing savings and efficiencies, but often also a loss of personal interaction." Mental health services have often become a kind of supermarket for services clients can access should they meet the requisite diagnostic criteria, and, even then, often for the McDonaldized services discussed earlier (Goodman 2016). Some readers might recall this fraught exchange over such managed services from the 1997 movie *As Good as It Gets*: "**Carol:** Fucking HMO [Health Management Organization] bastards pieces of shit! I'm sorry. **Doctor:** It's okay. Actually, I think that's their technical name" (Ziskin and Brooks 1997). Carol has just been turned down for medical services not covered by her HMO, but that she and her doctor agree are needed based on the circumstances she described. A whole cadre of mental health professionals have increasingly been pulled into public and private versions of a similar service-rationing delivery model, and arguably this has come with costs beyond those associated with professionals being paid.

The medicalizing story of counselling is not all bleak, of course, and someone has to pay for the services provided by counsellors. As the history of mental health shows, publicly as well as privately funded counselling in the second half of the twentieth century tended not to be so constrained by medicalizing discourse. People could go and talk to a professional counsellor when they could not find a receptive ear or help needed in their primary relationships—and yes, sometimes that might have led to a referral onto a psychiatric professional. Also, sometimes they only needed a single consultation (see Talmon 1990), or needed to be seen intermittently to enhance their physical and emotional well-being (Cummings and Sayama 2013). Frustratingly, for those who want to pull apart counselling and find the curative or life-enhancing things counsellors do, the best research repeatedly comes up with non-specific common factors related to the quality of the conversational relationship (Laska et al. 2014; Wampold and Imel 2015). What mostly matters, in other words, is a supportive relationship where clients can feel comfortable in being vulnerable when conversing about emotional experiences, while also finding focused ways to reflect upon and re-language those experiences in actionable ways (Tschacher et al. 2014). The added factor that Wampold and Imel (2015) bring is that good counselling addresses what clients want it to address.

Bringing this back to what I have become describing as conversational work in counselling, there clearly are no magic words or interventions to be administered, and this is especially the case for Greenberg's (2013) grey zone of "woe." There is a trajectory that sees people struggle with coping everyday life that puts them further along in developing psychopathology unless they get help (Zimmer-Gembeck and Skinner 2016). In many cases they do not have natural support systems, or the conversations needed require a step outside the hurly-burly of everyday life. Good conversational work remoralizes demoralized people (Frank 2004), and some of that happens through finding new ways of solving problems or coping, but other parts are harder to get a handle on. Counselling involves modest conversational work to collaboratively engage clients in finding new meanings and ways of moving forward when life gets tough (Wampold and Imel 2015), and medicalizing discourse might fit within such conversational work. There are many roads to Rome, as is often said.

Collaboration isn't about clients doing what is expected of them, it is about a relational process based on negotiating preferences or intentions regarding what moving on means for clients, and that might mean navigating what is unchangeable. For Wittgenstein's student, Elizabeth Anscombe (1957), intentions are actions under descriptions, and such descriptions, as those for addressing human concerns, are linguistic and often fluid. In medicalizing discourse, descriptions for concerns and what is to be done to address them are standardized and expertly diagnosed (i.e. fixed), for related forms of treatment. Intentions can, of course, be articulated in language. The tensions in counselling I have been describing can arise from rigidities in using any discourse, medicalizing as well others, such as that of the counsellor's favorite approach. In expertise-based professions, adherence to professional discourse is presumed to be how professional work gets done (Abbott 1988), but this often translates to monological exchanges of information and directives. Collaboration presumes more dialogical forms of interaction, a mutual negotiation of process and meaning toward an outcome that satisfies the client in ways that are ok for the counsellor (Anderson 1997). Such collaborations are not an "anything goes" professional encounter, but are critically reflective and generatively resourceful in helping clients address their concerns in ethical and accepted ways.

The dialogues of both counselling and medicine have long been recognized as having some give and take to them (Balint 1957), and medicalizing tensions are most likely to constrain this aspect of collaboration when adherence to standardized meanings and practices is required to guide what both client and counsellors are to say and hear. Variation will clash with standardization, goes a common medicalizing concern (Tanenbaum 2013). Medicalizing discourse in this sense runs counter prior to a common factors approach to counselling; and it thereby constrains the discursive awareness and resourcefulness clients and counsellors might use to address clients' concerns. Hence, I have been describing medicalizing tensions in counselling as those which compete for the words, evaluations, and conversational interactions of clients and counsellors. It relates to the Bakhtin (1981) comment raised in Chap. 8, about the word in any dialogue being "only half mine."

There is another way, however, that Bakhtin's words ring true and that rests with his unmodern conclusion; that there could be no final resting place for the word. There are only further responses, further words to be used. While medicalizing discourse offers a crystallization of contemporary wisdom on clients' medical symptoms and EBPs for addressing diagnosed disorders, my point throughout this book is that are further things to discuss beyond a medicalizing discourse—otherwise we can find ourselves back to Vico's ([1774] 2001) "linguistic poverty." For counsellors, whether it is through clients' expectations, or colleagues', the medicalizing discourse of DSM diagnoses and evidence-based treatments has acquired a cultural as well as institutional level of taken-for-granted common sense. So, it can feel odd to practice from other discourses, and to justify one's practice of alternative discourses, when medicalizing discourse has become so unquestioned as to be a default cultural discourse.

Afterthoughts

> We cannot escape words. We can only choose some of them: some of the gates, some of the dances, some of the music (Riikonen and Madan Smith 1997: 19).

As I bring my words to a close, I am reminded of John Shotter's (1993) book title, *The Cultural Politics of Everyday Life*. In a sense, I have been writing from such a premise throughout this book, and the medicalizing tensions I have been describing are about a form of everyday politics that plays out in the lives and practices of many a counsellor. Shotter, who died in the month I was concluding this book, introduced me to this sort of politics, as the book title implies Shotter (1993), but through a fascination for the possibilities of critically reflective and generative dialogue. In our conversations, John would dismiss medicalizing discourse, DSM discourse especially, as an abomination, and move quickly on to a different set of fluid but still highly responsive exigencies he saw as required of people to tackle important human concerns and aspirations in face-to-face dialogue. While speakers are always bringing discourses from outside their emergent relationship into their dialogues, some discourses offer more resources for helping the relationship move forward than do others. Moving forward, or going on, is an important phrase Shotter would frequently use, which he borrowed from Wittgenstein (1953), and relates to a very modest aim for dialogue, and especially for those occurring between client and counsellor.

Medicalizing discourse for counselling extends a tradition associated with Freud's "talking cure," and there will always be a need for psychiatric treatment. Counselling's aims have been modest and relationally focused on helping clients move on to get some version of what they came for, to find useful language they from which they can take acceptable new actions to address their concerns. Medicalizing discourse in counselling pre-establishes the meanings and conversational processes for those dialogues, purportedly legitimizing what concerns really are about, and how they should really be discussed. Medicalizing discourse and the tensions that come from its dominance need not constrain the possibilities for clients and counsellors to come up with new meanings and ways of talking together.

My hope in writing this book has been to invite critical reflection on a discourse that could easily become taken for granted in people's lives, let alone in counselling. Medicalizing discourse is a resource for improving one's well-being but not all of our concerns fall completely under the expansive term mental health. Counselling for the problems and difficulties that beset people will always be needed when the conversations they can have with close others come up short, or are not possible. May we stay discursively aware and resourceful in how we address our common and personal concerns.

References

Abbott, A. (1988). *The system of professions: An essay on the division of expert labor*. Chicago: University of Chicago Press.

Anderson, H. (1997). *Conversation, language, and possibilities: A postmodern approach to therapy*. New York: Basic Books.

Anscombe, G. E. M. (1957). *Intention*. Oxford: Basil Blackwell.

Aubrey, R. F. (1983). The odyssey of counseling and images of the future. *Personnel and Guidance Journal, 62*(2), 78–82.

Bakhtin, M. (1981). *The dialogic imagination: Four essays by M.M. Bakhtin*. Austin: University of Texas Press.

Balint, M. J. (1957). *The doctor, his patient, and the illness*. New York: International Universities Press.

Bowker, G. C., & Star, S. L. (2000). *Sorting things out: Classification and its consequences*. Cambridge, MA: MIT Press.

Busch, L. (2011). *Standards: Recipes for reality*. Cambridge, MA: MIT Press.

Chun, W. H. K. (2011). *Programmed visions: Software and memory*. Cambridge, MA: MIT Press.

Chun, W. H. K. (2016). *Updating to remain the same: Habitual new media.* Cambridge: MIT Press.

Chwalisz, K. (2003). Evidence-based practice: A framework for twenty-first century scientist-practitioner training. *The Counseling Psychologist, 31*(5), 497–528.

Collins, H., & Evans, R. (2009). *Rethinking expertise.* Chicago: University of Chicago Press.

Conrad, P. (2007). *The medicalization of society.* Baltimore: Johns Hopkins University Press.

Conti, R., Frank, R. G., & McGuire, T. G. (2004). Insuring mental health care in the age of managed care. In B. Lubotsky Levin, J. Petrila, & K. D. Hennessy (Eds.), *Mental health services: A public health perspective* (pp. 15–41). New York: Oxford University Press.

Cooper, M., & McLeod, J. (2011). *Pluralistic counselling and psychotherapy.* Thousand Oaks, CA: Sage.

Cummings, N., & Sayama, M. (2013). *Focused psychotherapy: A casebook of brief intermittent psychotherapy throughout the life cycle.* New York: Routledge.

Cushman, P. (1995). *Constructing the self, constructing America: A cultural history of psychotherapy.* Boston: Da Capo Press.

Danziger, K. (1997). *Naming the mind: How psychology found its language.* Thousand Oaks, CA: Sage.

De Vos, J. (2012). *Psychologisation in times of globalisation.* London: Routledge.

Dozois, D. J. (2013). Psychological treatments: Putting evidence into practice and practice into evidence. *Canadian Psychology/Psychologie Canadienne, 54*(1), 1–11.

Flores, F. (2012). *Conversations for action and collected essays: Instilling a culture of commitment in working relationships* (Kindle ed.). North Charleston: CreateSpace Independent Publishing Platform.

Foucault, M. (2008). *History of madness.* New York: Routledge.

Frances, A. (2013). *Saving normal: An insider's revolt against out-of-control psychiatric diagnosis, DSM-5, big pharma, and the medicalization of ordinary life.* New York: William Morrow.

Frankl, V. E. (2006). *Man's search for meaning.* Boston: Beacon Press.

Friedman, S. (Ed.). (1993). *The new language of change: Constructive collaboration in psychotherapy.* New York: Guilford Press.

Goodman, D. M. (2016). The mcdonaldization of psychotherapy: Processed foods, processed therapies, and economic class. *Theory & Psychology, 26*(1), 77–95.

Greenberg, G. (2013). *The book of woe: The DSM and the unmaking of psychiatry*. New York: Penguin.

Hacking, I. (1983). *Representing and intervening: Introductory topics in the philosophy of natural science*. Cambridge: Cambridge University Press.

Hacking, I. (1995). The looping effects of human kinds. In D. Sperber & A. J. Premack (Eds.), *Causal cognition* (pp. 351–383). Oxford: Oxford University Press.

Hook, D. (2007). *Foucault, psychology and the analytics of power*. London: Palgrave Macmillan.

Horwitz, A. V., & Wakefield, J. C. (2007). *The loss of sadness: How psychiatry transformed normal sorrow into depressive disorder*. New York: Oxford University Press.

Horwitz, A. V., & Wakefield, J. C. (2012). *All we have to fear: Psychiatry's transformation of natural anxieties into medical disorders*. New York: Oxford University Press.

Illouz, E. (2008). *Saving the modern soul: Therapy, emotions, and the culture of self-help*. Berkeley: University of California Press.

Insel, T. (2013). Post by former NIMH director Thomas Insel: Transforming diagnosis. Accessed November 18, 2016, from https://www.nimh.nih.gov/about/directors/thomas-insel/blog/2013/transforming-diagnosis.shtml.

Jutel, A. G. (2011). *Putting a name to it: Diagnosis in contemporary society*. Baltimore: Johns Hopkins University Press.

Kozart, M. F. (2002). Understanding efficacy in psychotherapy: An ethnomethodological perspective on the therapeutic alliance. *American Journal of Orthopsychiatry, 72*(2), 217–231.

Lakoff, G., & Johnson, M. (1980). *Metaphors we live by*. Chicago: University of Chicago Press.

Laska, K. M., Gurman, A. S., & Wampold, B. E. (2014). Expanding the lens of evidence-based practice in psychotherapy: A common factors perspective. *Psychotherapy (Chicago, IL), 51*(4): 467–481.

Latour, B. (1996). On interobjectivity. *Mind, Culture, and Activity, 3*(4), 228–245.

Lock, A., & Strong, T. (Eds.). (2012). *Discursive perspectives in therapeutic practice*. New York: Oxford University Press.

Miller, D., Acton, T. M., & Hedge, B. (1988). The worried well: their identification and management. *Journal of the Royal College of Physicians of London, 22*(3), 158–165.

Motes, P. S., & Smith, C. O. (2014). Systems of caregiving: The promotion of positive mental health outcomes in children and adolescents. In

R. C. Talley, G. L. Fricchione, & B. G. Druss (Eds.), *The challenges of mental health caregiving: Research, practice, policy* (pp. 103–121). New York: Springer.
Paré, D. (2013). *The practice of collaborative counseling and psychotherapy: Developing skills in culturally mindful helping*. Los Angeles: Sage.
Proctor, E. K., Landsverk, J., Aarons, G., Chambers, D., Glisson, C., & Mittman, B. (2009). Implementation research in mental health services: An emerging science with conceptual, methodological, and training challenges. *Administration and Policy in Mental Health and Mental Health Services Research, 36*(1), 24–34.
Rapley, M., Moncrieff, J., & Dillon, J. (2011). *De-medicalizing misery: Psychiatry, psychology and the human condition*. New York: Palgrave Macmillan.
Riikonen, E., & Madan Smith, G. (1997). *Re-imagining therapy: Living Conversations and relational knowing*. Thousand Oaks, CA: Sage.
Rorty, R. (1989). *Contingency, irony, and solidarity*. Cambridge: Cambridge University Press.
Shotter, J. (1993). *The cultural politics of everyday life*. Toronto: University of Toronto Press.
Steiner, C. (2012). *Automate this: How algorithms came to rule our world*. New York: Penguin.
Strong, T. (1993). DSM-IV and describing problems in family therapy. *Family Process, 32*, 249–253.
Strong, T. (1995). Clinical languages, clinical realities. *Human Systems: Journal of Systemic Consultation and Management, 6*(1), 53–65.
Strong, T., Ross, K. H., & Sesma-Vazquez, M. (2015). Counselling the (self?) diagnosed client: Generative and reflective conversations. *British Journal of Guidance and Counselling, 43*(5), 598–610.
Susskind, R., & Susskind, D. (2015). *The future of the professions: How technology will transform the work of human experts*. New York: Oxford University Press.
Szasz, T. (1961). *The myth of mental illness: Foundations of a theory of personal conduct*. New York: Hoeber-Harper.
Talmon, M. (1990). *Single session therapy: Maximizing the effect of the first (and often only) therapeutic encounter*. San Francisco: Jossey-Bass.
Tanenbaum, S. J. (2013). Reducing variation in health care: The rhetorical politics of a policy idea. *Journal of Health Politics, Policy and Law, 38*(1), 5–26.
Taylor, C. (1985). *Human agency and language: Philosophical papers 1*. Cambridge: Cambridge University Press.

Tschacher, W., Junghan, U. M., & Pfammatter, M. (2014). Towards a taxonomy of common factors in psychotherapy: Results of an expert survey. *Clinical Psychology & Psychotherapy, 21*(1), 82–96.

Turnbull, W. (2003). *Language in action: Psychological models of conversation*. New York: Psychology Press.

Tyler, L. E. (1953). *The work of the counselor*. New York: Appleton-Century Crofts.

Vico, G. ([1744] 2001). *The new science: Principles of the new science concerning the common nature of nations* (D. Marsh, Trans). New York: Penguin Books.

Wamboldt, M., Kaslow, N., & Reiss, D. (2015). Description of relational processes: Recent changes in DSM-5 and proposals for ICD-11. *Family Process, 54*(1), 6–16.

Wampold, B. E., & Imel, Z. E. (2015). *The great psychotherapy debate: The evidence for what makes psychotherapy work*. New York: Routledge.

Watzlawick, P., Weakland, J., & Fisch, R. (1974). *Change: Principles of problem formation and problem resolution*. New York: W.W. Norton.

Whitaker, R., & Cosgrove, L. (2015). *Psychiatry under the influence: Institutional corruption, social injury, and prescriptions for reform*. New York: Palgrave Macmillan.

Wittgenstein, L. (1953). *Philosophical investigations* (G. E. M. Anscombe, Trans.). Oxford: Basil Blackwell.

Zimmer-Gembeck, M. J., & Skinner, E. A. (2016). The development of coping: Implications for psychopathology and resilience. *Developmental Psychopathology, 4*(10), 1–61.

Ziskin, L. (Producer), & Brooks, J. L. (Director). (1997). *As good as it gets* [Motion picture]. Culver City: Tristar Pictures.

Further Reading

ACA (American Counseling Association). (2016). *What is counseling?* Accessed December 13, 2016 from https://www.counseling.org/about-us/about-aca.

Anderson, J. B. (2012). *Sick English: Medicalization in the English language* (Kindle DX version). Accessed from https://www.amazon.ca/Sick-English-Medicalization-Language-ebook/dp/B00AEH3BEQ.

Archer, S. T. (2015). *U.S. patent no. US9155891 B2*. Mountain view: Neuropace, Inc. Accessed December 6, 2016, from https://www.google.com/patents/US9155891.

Audet, C., & Paré, D. A. (Eds.). (2017). *Social justice and counselling*. New York: Routledge.

Bauman, Z. (2000). *Liquid modernity*. Malden: Blackwell.

Binet, A. S. T. (1916). *The development of intelligence in children: The binet-simon scale* (E. S. Kite, Trans.). Publications of the Training School at Vineland New Jersey Department of Research No. 11. Baltimore: Williams & Wilkins.

Binkley, S. (2011). Psychological life as enterprise: Social practice and the government of neo-liberal interiority. *History of the Human Sciences, 24*(3), 83–102.

Bohart, A. C., & Tallman, K. (1996). The active client: Therapy as self-help. *Journal of Humanistic Psychology, 36*(3), 7–30.

Bordin, E. S. (1950). Counseling methods: Therapy. *Annual Review of Psychology, 1*(1), 267–276.

T. Strong, *Medicalizing Counselling*, Palgrave Studies in the Theory and History of Psychology, DOI 10.1007/978-3-319-56699-3

Brinkmann, S. (2016). *Diagnostic cultures: A cultural approach to the pathologization of modern life*. London: Routledge.

Brown, L. S. (2006). Still subversive after all these years: The relevance of feminist therapy in the age of evidence-based practice. *Psychology of Women Quarterly, 30*(1), 15–24.

Burkeman, O. (2016, December 22). Why time management is ruining our lives. *The Guardian*. Accessed December 25, 2016, from https://www.theguardian.com/technology/2016/dec/22/why-time-management-is-ruining-our-lives?CMP=share_btn_fb.

Butler, J. (1997). *The psychic life of power: Theories in subjection*. Stanford: Stanford University Press.

Carter, E. A., & McGoldrick, M. (Eds.). (1980). *The changing family life cycle: A framework for family therapy*. New York: Gardner Press.

CCPA (Canadian Counselling and Psychotherapy Association). (2016). *The profession*. Accessed December 13, 2016, from https://www.ccpa-accp.ca/profession/.

Chambless, D. L., Sanderson, W. C., Shoham, V., et al. (1996). An update on empirically validated therapies. *Clinical Psychology, 49*(2), 5–18.

Chung, R. C., & Bemak, F. (2012). *Social justice counseling: The next steps beyond multiculturalism*. Thousand Oaks, CA: Sage.

Coffey, R. M., Buck, J. A., Kassed, C. A., Dilonardo, J., Carol Forhan, M. B. A., Marder, W. D., et al. (2008). Transforming mental health and substance abuse data systems in the United States. *Psychiatric Services, 59*(11), 1257–1263.

CPA (Canadian Psychological Association). (2016). *Definition of counselling psychology*. Accessed December 13, 2016, from http://www.cpa.ca/aboutcpa/cpasections/counsellingpsychology.

Cushman, P. (1990). Why the self is empty: Toward a historically situated psychology. *American Psychologist, 45*(5), 599–611.

Daniels, J. A., & Larson, L. M. (2001). The impact of performance feedback on counseling self-efficacy and counselor anxiety. *Counselor Education and Supervision, 41*(2), 120–130.

Dean, M. (2013). *The signature of power: Sovereignty, governmentality and biopolitics*. London: Sage.

DeFehr, J. N. (2016). Inventing mental health first aid: The problem of psychocentrism. *Studies in Social Justice, 10*(1), 18–35.

Deleuze, G., & Guattari, F. (1987). *A thousand plateaus: Capitalism and schizophrenia*. London: Continuum.

Derrida, J. (1976). *Of grammatology* (G. C. Spivak, Trans.). Baltimore: Johns Hopkins University Press.

Dhand, R. (2016). Creating a cultural analysis tool for the implementation of Ontario's civil mental health laws. *International Journal of Law and Psychiatry, 45*, 25–42.

Dow Schüll, N. (2012). *Addiction by design: Machine gambling in Las Vegas*. Princeton: Princeton University Press.

Ebeling, M. (2011). 'Get with the program!' Pharmaceutical marketing, symptom checklists and self-diagnosis. *Social Science & Medicine, 73*(6), 825–832.

Ehrenreich, B. (2009). *Bright-sided: How the relentless promotion of positive thinking has undermined America*. New York: Metropolitan Books.

Eisenberg, D., Downs, M. F., Golberstein, E., & Zivin, K. (2009). Stigma and help seeking for mental health among college students. *Medical Care Research and Review, 66*(5), 522–541.

Foucault, M. (1988). Technologies of the self. In L. H. Marin, H. Gutman, & P. H. Hutton (Eds.), *Technologies of the self: A seminar with Michel Foucault* (pp. 16–49). Amherst, MA: University of Massachusetts Press.

Foucault, M. (1990). *The history of sexuality*, Vol. 1: *An Introduction*. New York: Random House.

Foucault, M. (2005). *The hermeneutics of the subject: Lectures at the Collège de France, 1981–1982*. New York: Picador.

Foucault, M. (2010). *The government of self and others: Lectures at the Collège de France, 1982–1983*. New York: Picador.

Frank, A. W. (1995). *The wounded storyteller: Body, illness, and ethics*. Chicago: University of Chicago Press.

Frank, A. W. (2004). *The renewal of generosity: Illness, medicine, and how to live*. Chicago: University of Chicago Press.

Giles, D. C. (2014). 'DSM-V is taking away our identity': The reaction of the online community to the proposed changes in the diagnosis of Asperger's disorder. *Health, 18*(2), 179.

Grohol, J. (2016). Symptoms and treatments of mental disorders. *Psych Central*. Accessed November 28, 2016, from http://psychcentral.com/disorders/.

Guignon, C. (2004). *On being authentic*. New York: Routledge.

Hansen, J. T. (2007). Should counseling be considered a health care profession? Critical thoughts on the transition to a health care ideology. *Journal of Counseling & Development, 85*(3), 286–293.

Haslam, N., & Kvaale, E. P. (2015). Biogenetic explanations of mental disorder: The mixed-blessings model. *Current Directions in Psychological Science, 24*(5), 399–404.

Hill, N. (1937). *Think and grow rich*. Cleveland, OH: The Ralston Publishing Company.

House, R. (2010). *In, against and beyond therapy: Critical essays toward a "Post-professional" era*. Ross-on-Wye: PCCS Books.

Hoyt, K. B. (1962). Guidance: A constellation of services. *Personnel and Guidance Journal, 40*(8), 690–697.

Huxley, A. (1932). *Brave new world*. New York: Harper & Brothers.

Illouz, E. (2003). *Oprah Winfrey and the glamour of misery: An essay on popular culture*. New York: Columbia University Press.

Ingold, T. (2007). *Lines: A brief history*. New York: Routledge.

Ingold, T. (2015). *The life of lines*. New York: Routledge.

Ivey, A. E., Ivey, M. B., & Simek-Morgan, L. (1993). *Counseling and psychotherapy: Integrating skills, theory, and practice* (3rd ed.). Englewood Cliffs, NJ: Prentice Hall.

Jorm, A. F. (2000). Mental health literacy: Public knowledge and beliefs about mental disorders. *British Journal of Psychiatry, 177*(5), 396–401.

Keohane, K., & Petersen, A. (Eds.). (2013). *The social pathologies of contemporary civilization*. New York: Routledge.

Kramer, P. D. (2016). *Ordinarily well: The case for antidepressants*. New York: Farrar, Straus & Giroux.

Krans, B. (2016, May 9). *The 17 best depression blogs of 2016*. Accessed November 28, 2016, from http://www.healthline.com/health/depression/best-blogs-of-the-year#3.

Lazzarato, M. (2014). *Signs and machines: Capitalism and the production of capitalism*. Los Angeles: Semiotext(e).

Lenny, A. (2009). *The worried well*. Accessed from http://www.cfpc.ca/ProjectAssets/Templates/Resource.aspx?id=4489.

Lunau, K. (2012). *The mental health crisis on campus*. Accessed November 30, 2016, from http://www.macleans.ca/education/uniandcollege/the-mental-health-crisis-on-campus/.

Mallinckrodt, B., & Nelson, M. L. (1991). Counselor training level and the formation of the psychotherapeutic working alliance. *Journal of Counseling Psychology, 38*(2), 133–138.

Martin, L., Turcotte, M., Matte, L., & Shepard, B. (2013). The counselling and psychotherapy profession in Canada: Regulatory processes and current status. *British Journal of Guidance & Counselling, 41*(1), 46–57.

McKinlay, A., & Taylor, P. (2014). *Foucault, governmentality, and organization.* New York: Routledge.

Menne, J. M. (1975). A comprehensive set of counselor competencies. *Journal of Counseling Psychology, 22*(6), 547–553.

Miller, D., Acton, T. M., & Hedge, B. (1988). The worried well: Their identification and management. *Journal of the Royal College of Physicians of London, 22*(3), 158–165.

Miller, I. (1998, June). *Eleven unethical managed care practices every patient should know about.* Accessed December 29, 2016, from http://www.oregoncounseling.org/Consumer/ElevenDeceptivePrinciples.htm#5.%20Practicing%20outside%20of%20a%20professional%27s%20area%20of%20competence.

Miller, P., & Rose, N. (2008). *Governing the present: Administering economic, social and personal life.* Cambridge: Polity Press.

Moncrieff, J. (2008). *The myth of the chemical cure: A critique of psychiatric drug treatment.* New York: Palgrave MacMillan.

Morey, M. E., Arora, P., & Stark, K. D. (2015). Multiple-stage screening of youth depression in schools. *Psychology in the Schools, 52*(8), 800–814.

Moss, P., & Teghtsoonian, K. (2008). *Contesting illness: Processes and practices.* Toronto: University of Toronto Press.

Murgia, M. (2016, June 21). Dr Google will see you now: New health symptom checker takes on GPs. *The Telegraph.* Accessed November 28, 2016, from http://www.telegraph.co.uk/technology/2016/06/21/dr-google-will-see-you-now-new-health-symptom-checker-takes-on-g/.

Murphy, C. (2007, September 19). Dealing with the worried well. *BBC News.* Accessed November 18, 2016, from http://news.bbc.co.uk/2/hi/health/7001436.stm.

Murray, B. (2003). A brief history of RxP. Accessed November 25, 2016, from http://www.apa.org/monitor/oct03/rxp.aspx.

Nesi, J., & Prinstein, M. J. (2015). Using social media for social comparison and feedback-seeking: Gender and popularity moderate associations with depressive symptoms. *Journal of Abnormal Child Psychology, 43*(8), 1427–1438.

Neuer Colburn, A. A., Grothaus, T., Hays, D. G., & Milliken, T. (2016). A delphi study and initial validation of counselor supervision competencies. *Counselor Education and Supervision, 55*(1), 2–15.

OED. (2015). *Psychotherapy.* Accessed May 23, 2015, from http://www.oed.com/view/Entry/153946?rskey=jNoItF&result=1.

Padamsee, T. J. (2011). The pharmaceutical corporation and the 'good work' of managing women's bodies. *Social Science & Medicine, 72*(8), 1342–1350.

Parikh, S. V. (2015). Improving access to psychosocial treatments: Integrating patient, provider, and systems approaches. *Canadian Journal of Psychiatry, 60*(6), 242–244.

Parker, I. (Ed.). (2015). *Handbook of critical psychology*. New York: Routledge.

Peale, N. V. (1952). *The power of positive thinking and the amazing results of positive thinking*. New York: Prentice Hall.

Pinder, C. C., & Bourgeois, V. W. (1982). Controlling tropes in administrative science. *Administrative Science Quarterly, 27*(4), 641.

Prime Minister's Office. (2008, May 7). *Clarifying statement to the government's response to the psychotherapy e-petition*. Government of the United Kingdom. Accessed from http://www.number10.gov.uk/Page15454.

Prince, M. J. (2008). Claiming a disability benefit as contesting social citizenship. In P. Moss & K. Teghtsoonian (Eds.), *Contesting illness: Processes and practice* (pp. 28–46). Toronto: University of Toronto Press.

Ravenscroft, I. (2016, August 16). Folk psychology as theory. *Stanford Encyclopedia of Philosophy*. Accessed November 28, 2016, from http://plato.stanford.edu/entries/folkpsych-theory/.

Rich, E., & Miah, A. (2017). Mobile, wearable and ingestible health technologies: Towards a critical research agenda. *Health Sociology Review, 26*(1), 84–97.

Romelli, K., Frigerio, A., & Colombo, M. (2016). DSM over time: From legitimisation of authority to hegemony. *Biosocieties, 11*(1), 1–21.

Rose, N. (1997). *Inventing our selves: Psychology, power, and personhood*. Cambridge: Cambridge University Press.

Rosenbaum, P. J., & Liebert, H. (2015). Reframing the conversation on college student mental health. *Journal of College Student Psychotherapy, 29*(3), 179–196.

Sabin, J. E., & Daniels, N. (1994). Determining 'medical necessity' in mental health practice. *The Hastings Center Report, 24*(6), 5–13.

Sflakidou, S., & Kefalopoulou, M. (2015). The person-centred approach as an ideological discourse: A discourse analysis of person-centred counsellors' accounts on their way of being. *European Journal of Psychotherapy & Counselling, 17*(2), 179.

Sinacola, R. S., & Peters-Strickland, T. S. (2011). *Basic psychopharmacology for counselors and psychotherapists* (2nd ed.). Boston: Pearson.

Slater, L. (1998). *Prozac diary*. New York: Penguin Books.

Smith, A. J., & Siegel, R. F. (1985). Feminist therapy: Redefining power for the powerless. In L. E. A. Walker & L. B. Rosewater (Eds.), *Handbook of feminist therapy: Women's issues in psychotherapy* (pp. 13–21). New York: Springer.

Steers, M. N., Wickham, R. E., & Acitelli, L. K. (2014). Seeing everyone else's highlight reels: How Facebook usage is linked to depressive symptoms. *Journal of Social and Clinical Psychology, 33*(8), 701–731.

Stewart, D. W., Walker, J. R., Beatie, B., Reynolds, K. A., Hahlweg, K., Leonhart, M., et al. (2014). Postsecondary students' information needs and pathways for help with stress, anxiety, and depression/Les besoins d'information des étudiants postsecondaires et les parcours conçus pour réduire le stress, l'anxiété, et la dépression. *Canadian Journal of Counselling and Psychotherapy (Online), 48*(3), 356–374.

Strong, T. (2011). Approaching problem gambling with a discursive sensibility. *Journal of Gambling Issues, 25,* 68–87.

Strong, T. (2014). Brief therapy and the DSM: 13 possible conversational tensions. *Journal of Brief Therapy, 9*(1–2), 1–12.

Strong, T. (2015). Diagnoses, relational processes and resourceful dialogues: Tensions for families and family therapy. *Family Process, 54,* 518–532.

Super, D. E. (1953). A theory of vocational development. *American Psychologist, 8*(5), 185–190.

Swan, E. (2010). *Worked up selves: Personal development workers, self-work and therapeutic cultures.* New York: Palgrave Macmillan.

Taylor, C. (1989). *Sources of the self: The making of the modern identity.* Cambridge, MA: Harvard University Press.

Thompson, R. (2012). Screwed up, but working on it: (Dis)ordering the self through e-stories. *Narrative Inquiry, 22*(1), 86–104.

Toscano, A., & Kinkle, J. (2015). *Cartographies of the absolute: An aesthetics of the economy for the twenty-first century.* London: Zero Books.

TRC (Truth and Reconciliation Commission of Canada). (2015). *TRC findings.* Accessed November 28, 2016, from http://www.trc.ca/websites/trcinstitution/index.php?p=890.

Turner, B. S. (2006). *Vulnerability and human rights.* Philadelphia: Penn State University Press.

University of Calgary. (2015). *Campus mental health strategy.* Accesed from http://ucalgary.ca/provost/files/provost/15-unv-018-mental_health_strategy_final.pdf.

Vander Schee, C. (2007). The politics of health as a school-sponsored ethic: Foucault, neoliberalism, and the unhealthy employee. *Educational Policy, 22*(6), 854–874.

Walters, W. (2012). *Governmentality: Critical encounters*. New York: Routledge.
Washington, H. A. (2016). *Infectious madness: The surprising science of how we "catch" mental illness*. New York: Little, Brown & Company.
Weingarten, K. (1998). The small and the ordinary: The daily practice of a postmodern narrative therapy. *Family Process, 37*(1), 3–15.
Wessler, R. L., & Hankin-Wessler, S. W. (1989). Nonconscious algorithms in cognitive and affective processes. *Journal of Cognitive Psychotherapy, 3*(4), 243–254.
White, M. (1995). *Re-authoring live: Interviews and essays*. Adelaide: Dulwich Centre.
WHO (World Health Organization). (2003). *WHO definition of health*. Accessed November 28, 2016, from http://www.who.int/about/definition/en/print.html.
Wikipedia. (2016a). *List of counseling topics*. Accessed November 21, 2016, from https://en.wikipedia.org/wiki/List_of_counseling_topics.
Wikipedia. (2016b). *Mental health professional*. Accessed November 1, 2016, from https://en.wikipedia.org/wiki/Mental_health_professional.
Wikipedia. (2016c). *Psychotherapy*. Accessed November 21, 2016, from https://en.wikipedia.org/wiki/Psychotherapy.
Worden, J. W. (1991). *Grief counseling and grief therapy* (2nd ed.). New York: Springer.

Index

T. Strong, *Medicalizing Counselling*, Palgrave Studies in the Theory and History of Psychology, DOI 10.1007/978-3-319-56699-3

Q

R

Printed by Printforce, the Netherlands